When Sex Becomes Intimate

How Sexuality Changes As Your Relationship Deepens

Krishnananda Trobe, MD and Amana Trobe

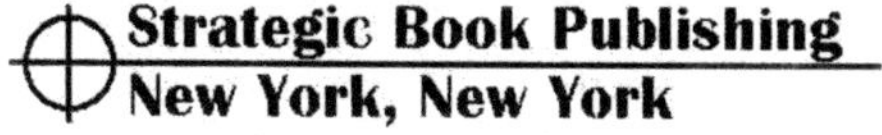

Strategic Book Publishing
An imprint of Writers Literary & Publishing Services, Inc.
845 Third Avenue, 6th Floor – 6016
New York, NY 10022
www.strategicbookpublishing.com

ISBN: 978-1-934925-79-9/SKU 1-934925-79-9

Printed in the United States of America

Cover Design by Anugito Sedona, Arizona - artlinegraphics.com

Cover Painting by Michael Colpitts Sedona, Arizona - artfulceramics.com (paintings)

For information about Krishnananda and Amana - www.learningloveseminars.com

Table Of Contents

Introduction
Keeping Our Sex Life Alive

For many years, we've been leading workshops in which we teach people how to love — themselves and another. One of the topics that very often arises, particularly for couples that have been together for some time, is how to keep their sexuality alive. Couples notice that often the longer they are together; the more difficult it is to maintain the same interest in making love. Life's stresses, familiarity, and lack of communication may wear away at their desire to make love. Perhaps they long for those early days when they couldn't wait to jump into bed and have hot, passionate sex. Or maybe they long for a deeper way to connect through lovemaking, but it doesn't happen.

Sex changes as intimacy deepens. But unless you appreciate and learn how to adjust to the change, you may not know how to deal with it. Sex is a significant aspect of togetherness; if it fades, it can threaten the relationship. And if it fades, you may easily get restless or resentful. You may begin having affairs or become resigned, bitter and/or depressed. Or you may find yourself drawn to other things like the computer, television, work, sports or other hobbies, and not take the time to connect with your partner.

When you come closer to someone, you become more vulnerable. That vulnerability usually also means increased fears and insecurities. Sex can bring up feelings of vulnerability more strongly than just about any experience in your life. Most of us can remember painful and humiliating or even frightening moments related to our sexuality. And sometimes you may not know that you're traumatized sexually, but your body is showing fear without even knowing it. It is frozen fear, what we call "shock" that can cause sexual dysfunction. If you've not explored, understood or accepted your fears and insecurities, particular in connection to your sexuality, you may not know what to do or even what they are when they arise. You may feel that something is wrong with you or with the relationship. You may try to compensate for the fears by pushing yourself in sex in a way that doesn't feel right.

When we're feeling frightened or insecure while making love, it drastically affects how we respond and also the way we want to make love. In lovemaking, especially as we come closer to another person, it becomes more and more crucial to feel safe.

It's natural and even healthy that the kind of excitement that was present in the honeymoon period of the relationship may fade. Excitement may happen easily when you are making love to someone you have just met. But if it diminishes with time, you may try to keep the excitement going one way or another. These methods become increasingly artificial and contrived. The solution to this problem is to discover something deeper and more sustaining that eventually replaces your need for perpetual excitement.

Excitement cannot be the sustaining force in the sexuality of a long-term relationship.

As we sat down to write this book, we'd been together for fourteen years. We met originally in India where we were both practicing meditation and living in a spiritual commune. One of the aspects of the commune was an active program of growth workshops. When we first got together as a couple, we decided to take a two-week tantra (sexuality) workshop. The course was teaching a way of integrating meditation and sexuality in a specific approach and technique of lovemaking that attracted us. (We'll be describing this approach in some detail in a later chapter.)

At the time we took this workshop, I (Krish) was also seeking a change in the way I'd been making love. One reason was that I was seeking deeper, more loving and more meditative connecting in sex. But there was another reason. In my lovemaking, I was afraid of coming too fast when my partner or I got excited. I felt intense shame when it happened and I couldn't really relax because of this fear. The method we learned stressed connection rather than performance and taught lovemaking in such a relaxed, non-doing way that something inside of me deeply relaxed. I noticed that when I took the time to relax and became more focused on the connection rather than on the excitement of lovemaking, something changed for me. The absence of pressure and expectations has helped me to recover from my insecurity and dysfunction. In fact, we have found that this absence of pressure and demands in sex is one of the most important ingredients that allow couples to keep their love and sex life alive.

It was also very nourishing for me (Amana) to discover that lovemaking can be so relaxing and deeply satisfying without doing anything. I found that just by connecting and allowing the bodies and the energies to melt, something much deeper happens than can happen with a lot of doing. In fact this workshop prepared our relationship for a different way of being together, where lovemaking is not about excitement or sexual satisfaction but rather about connecting.

In our own sexual relationship, we continue to face challenges of encountering fears and insecurities and working through them. What's more, in just about any deep relationship, each person's wounds have a way of triggering the wounds of the other. And each person has to confront deeply unconscious and automatic ways that he or she pushes the other person away and hides — and then retreats from making love. In our own case, Krish's fears of being overwhelmed by a powerful woman and then going into shock (originating from a strong and overpowering mother) can run a collision course with Amana's experience of her man's not being present (originating from an alcoholic father who escaped into addiction and eventually killed himself.) With love and awareness, we have managed to deal with this dynamic in a creative way.

As we go deeper into intimacy, we need to understand how fear, shame, shock and self-doubt affect our sexuality. We need to learn how to communicate our experience in sex, particularly our vulnerabilities. And, most likely, our sexuality may need to adjust and incorporate our increased vulnerability.

But there's more to a healthy sexual relationship for a long-term couple than learning to make sensitive love. You also have to keep your emotional house clean and work toward deepening the love between you. There were twelve couples that took the workshop together with us. But as far as we know, of the twelve, we're the only couple that survived. And the reason these relationships ended, for the most part, was because unresolved emotional conflicts tore apart the fiber of their love.

We have been able to keep *our* love and our sexuality very much alive partly because we have made it a priority from the beginning to deal with anything that creates distance and hurt between us. Our intimacy is such that we can feel it whenever something disturbs our closeness. We have learned, from working with ourselves, that when we feel triggered, reactive or distant from each other, it is mostly because some early wound has been opened which we are still sensitive about. Or, it can be because we're feeling stressed and we take out that stress on the other person.

Sex can be the first causality of stress that is not dealt with and unresolved conflicts. You may have no idea that you're heading into an emotional minefield when you become close to someone. You just want things to flow harmoniously and conflict-free as they may have done in the early days of your togetherness. Love is not like that. Love brings up your unresolved wounds, your fears of invasion and abandonment, your dependency, your fears of losing yourself in the other person, your expectations, and your buried resentments toward the opposite sex.

We all need tools and understanding to navigate through all the emotional issues that come up. We need to know what is being triggered, how to deal with it inside — and, above all, how to communicate. Most of us didn't have much experience with learning these lessons before we found ourselves in a relationship. We didn't go to "intimacy school" before falling in love.

What's more, most of the time your reactions and disturbances may have little or nothing to do with the other person. They have to do with a lack of inner space in the moment and feeling overwhelmed by life. When you get provoked or stressed, often all you want to do is blame someone or something or find someone or something to make you feel better. And when you lack inner space, the smallest thing that the other person does or any kind of life stressor, disappointment or frustration can easily provoke your agitation and fears and cause you to react. When you're reacting *toward* each other, sex suffers.

Behind our conflicts, resentments and hurt is fear and pain. It is a big part of the inner world of our vulnerability.. Yet vulnerability is also the doorway to the most profound and precious parts of ourselves, to the treasures of our soul and to the heart of intimacy.

This is not a tantra book. It does not deal with teaching new and different ways of making love in order to improve orgasm or using sex to reach ecstatic states. That is not our expertise, and there are many excellent books that deal with these topics. In this book, we provide a roadmap for bringing sex and vulnerability together so that it can become a way of deepening and enriching intimacy. Too often, relationships and sex falter because of a lack of understanding of our underlying sensitivities and a lack of the tools to communicate and resolve hurts and resentments. It's our sincere hope that we can provide concrete ways to deal with these issues in these pages. In the course of the book, we give examples from our own life and also from those of people we have worked with. Naturally, to protect the confidentiality of those we discuss, we either omit names or change the names of those we discuss.

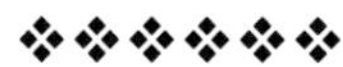

Part 1

An Overview —
A Model for Sex and Intimacy

Chapter 1
"Am I Making Love in the Right Way for Me?" Levels of Sexual Experience

Adrian and Lisa have been together for seven years. They're having trouble in their sex life because Adrian feels that Lisa is not allowing him to be alive, uninhibited and spontaneous in their lovemaking, while Lisa feels that he's moving too fast, and his sexual intensity frightens her. In the moments that her fear comes up and she tells him that he needs to be more sensitive to her, he sees and feels his mother who was always repressed and guilty about her own sexuality and was not supportive of his sexuality either. For Lisa, it is a different story. She experienced sexual abuse as a child that she only recently discovered and now feels fear even at the thought of making love. Finding a way for them to be sensitive to each other and to allow their sexuality to develop inclusive of their wounds has taken some work.

Here is an excerpt from an argument they had in one of their sessions with us:

Adrian: "When we make love, I hate it when you hold me back. It makes me feel controlled and even castrated."

Lisa: "Adrian, I don't mean to hold you back. But when you come at me with this kind of male energy, my body contracts."

Adrian: "It never used to be like this. You used to love it when I turned you on."

Lisa: " I know, but that was in the beginning. Now it's different. I like your intensity and your maleness, but for some reason, when we are making love, it becomes too much. And when you start to move so fast inside of me, I get scared."

Adrian: "You're just afraid of energy because you can't let go of control."

Lisa: "And you're afraid of being vulnerable."

And at this point, communication breaks down and they are in a stalemate.

This example brings up important issues that concern couples who have been together for some time. In the beginning of a relationship, the novelty of the situation often allows you to have compatibility and a harmony. But that can change as you go deeper. We would like to take a little time now to give you a model. We presented this model in an earlier book, *Face to Face With Fear — A Journey From Fear to Freedom* to help people to understand their inner world and to help them understand the journey of learning love. It's a drawing of three circles representing your emotional and spiritual make-up — a large circle with a smaller one inside and an even smaller one inside the second circle.

The outer ring represents your layer of protection and defenses — your strategies of control, withdrawal, fight, manipulation, possessiveness, demand, expectations, giving up, mentalizing, your addictions to substances, work, food, sex — all the ways you may distract yourself from feeling.

The middle ring represents your wounded vulnerability — basically your fears and insecurities. It includes your fear of getting close to someone, your fears of abandonment or engulfment, of invasion and disrespect, your fear of expressing yourself, of confronting someone or being honest, of being humiliated, judged or criticized, or of being alone. It is in this layer that you carry your hurts and the body memory of earlier traumas. It is the space of your wounded innocence and trust, your longings for love but also your fears of opening and exposing your vulnerability.

The inner circle represents your essence — your natural aliveness, sensitivity, joy, free sexuality, strength, clarity, silence, lovingness and wisdom. Most of us have had glimpses of this space either in meditation, lovemaking, sports, while in nature or with psychedelic drugs, but we rarely live in our essence most of the time. Naturally, there is a longing to have bigger tastes of this state which can drive you to becoming dependent on what gives you the glimpse — i.e. drugs, extreme sports, sex etc.

When you first begin a relationship, any relationship but especially a sexual one, you will often meet in the essential layer. That's why things can go so smoothly at first. Your energy is high, you feel happy to have met someone you can relate with and your sexuality might be very exciting and even ecstatic. But this "honeymoon" space rarely lasts. With time, disappointments and frustrations arise and earlier wounds also get triggered. Now, one or both of you are experiencing the middle (wounded) layer. Rather than feel and work through these fears and hurts, you normally move directly into your outer (protection) layer. The honeymoon is over.

This model also helps you understand how your sexuality changes as intimacy deepens. We describe these changes as three distinct levels of sexual experience. They are not linear, nor is one "higher" or "better" than another. They are just different.

These levels also describe an inner journey and the natural progression of two people growing in intimacy and love. Our spiritual master paid a lot of attention to sexuality. He had the insight that spiritual traditions which were repressive of sex only led to false morality, aggression, repression, guilt and sickness. He taught that if we allowed ourselves to explore our sexuality freely, we would naturally long for and seek out a sexuality that would became more focused on connection and meditation. We have both been deeply inspired by this approach. We have lived it and watched our own transition precisely in the way that he described. Before we met, both us had times in our lives when we explored our sexuality. By the time we came together, we felt we "had done that and lived that" and were seeking something deeper and more nourishing.

"Level One Sex"

"Level one sex" is essentially about energy, passion and excitement. It is a wonderful experience of arousal and exploration. It is focused on pleasure and orgasm, on deepening satisfaction, and on learning how to pleasure yourself as well as to pleasure the other person. "Level one sex" is also concerned with overcoming inhibitions and allowing your sexuality to become free of the repressions with which many of us were conditioned. It is learning to enjoy your body and the body of the other person without guilt. It is learning to explore and enjoy different ways of making love with variety and adventure. It may even include a period of making love with different partners.

When you're enjoying sex without repression, you feel alive and vital. If you've missed a period in your life when you were able to explore your sexuality, you might easily long for it. Repressive conditioning may have caused you to miss these experiences. But at some point, you may have started to question this repressive conditioning. Then "forbidden" thoughts may start to creep into the mind — fantasies of having wild sexual adventures, finding yourself surfing the Internet, looking at attractive men or women, or feeling disconnected in your marriage — all because you are missing "level one sex." We encounter many situations such as this in our work. Often the root of a couple's problems is that one or both are longing for some good "level one sex" that they never had.

It is not uncommon for people who have settled into a comfortable and secure domestic life with each other to later discover that they've never explored their sexuality. If both partners are willing, they can find support in workshops or from a therapist or guide to explore this together. Often, though, this becomes the reason that long-term couples separate because there is not enough mutual insight about the need to heal from the guilt and repression surrounding sex.

Most of us hunger and fantasize about having sex that is deeply pleasurable, passionate and orgasmic. If we've never lived it out, we may find ourselves longing for it for much of our life. And because so many of us have been conditioned with all kinds of guilt and repressive messages about sex, the desire for this kind of sex can be like a volcano inside waiting to erupt.

There is a downside to what we call "level one sex." When your focus is on pleasure and orgasm, you can run into trouble when vulnerability arises. Vulnerability can cause fear, contraction and dysfunction and you may not want anything to interfere with the free expression of your sexuality. So, to hold down your vulnerability, you become compensated. You may push yourself to get more pleasure or to please your partner or push yourself to have stronger orgasms, harder erections or longer-lasting lovemaking. Then, your sexuality can easily become disconnected.

Compensating behaviors can include focusing on performance and on orgasm, feeling compelled to perform to satisfy your own expectations or those of the other person, becoming driven, impatient and demanding sexually. It can show itself in obsessive thinking and fantasizing. One client admitted openly to us that if he allowed himself to feel his insecurities, he could not perform adequately. He would either come too fast or would lose his erection. He was terrified that his partner would judge him and find someone else. Another client told us that she never shared her fears with her partner because "if he knew how frightened I was, he wouldn't be attracted to me anymore."

The biggest problem with "level one sex" is that when you resist feeling your vulnerability, you can find yourself drawn to what we call "objective sex." In "objective sex," you are not making deep intimate contact with your partner; you are focused on the excitement and the stimulation. "Objective sex" allows you to be stimulated and excited without having to deal with what can become troublesome insecurities and fears lurking in the unconscious. The attraction of "objective sex," as we will discuss in a later chapter, is the reason that sex can become addictive and one reason that so many people are attracted to pornography.

> *In short, "level one sex" is fun, exciting and even ecstatic. But if we are attached to the intensity and do not allow our fears and insecurities to arise, with time and deeper closeness, it can lead to compensation and addiction.*

"Level Two Sex"

When you begin to become more vulnerable while making love, you enter into what we call, "level two sex." You begin to feel the need for something different in your lovemaking. One reason can be that you long for a deeper connection with your partner and you feel dissatisfied with the way you've been making love up to now. But more frequently, insecurity and fear may be surfacing and it is affecting your sexuality. You may begin to experience dysfunctions, pain, contractions, and even unclear memories of earlier traumas. At a certain point, you can no longer hide it or run away from it. And then, as we have mentioned earlier, you may want to avoid sex or try to compensate to push aside the fear or insecurity that is coming up.

> *We often compensate or avoid sex so as not to enter into "level two" or what we call the "vulnerability layer."*

Some of you may find that you are in "level two" even from the beginning of a sexual relationship. For others, it develops as you get closer to another person. As you become more vulnerable, you can no longer defend yourself so easily from prior painful experiences that still affect your body, your sexuality and your nervous system. When this happens, symptoms of trauma start to show themselves more readily. Many clients with whom we've worked have reported that after being in a relationship for some time, they began to discover how frightened and insecure they were while making love. Others are not aware of the fear and insecurity inside but they are troubled by dysfunctions that were not there in the beginning.

There are some challenges in "level two sex." For one, you may miss the uncomplicated sexual high of "level one." You may long for the "good old days" when you could perform sexually without it being complicated by your fear and insecurities. You may even try to manipulate your sexuality so that you don't have to feel so vulnerable. Furthermore, you may find yourself with a partner who is impatient with your insecurities and fears. You may also not understand or know how to communicate when fears and insecurities arise. Often, you may not even be aware that you are afraid or ashamed, but your body knows and will fail to respond or function the way you would like it to. For a woman, this may show itself by not feeling excitement, not being able to have an orgasm, vaginal infections or dryness, and pelvic or bladder infections. For a man, it can show as genital pain, not getting an erection, or premature ejaculation. For both, it can also show itself in fantasies or by spacing out while making love.

> *We cannot fight with our vulnerability. If fear and insecurity are arising in connection to sex, they need to be dealt with. It is not going to go away. Sex may have been one of our most favorite ways of avoiding deeper inner spaces, but if the body is reacting by not functioning the way we would like it to we may no longer have this as an avenue of escape.*

Problems can arise when one person is in "level two" and beginning to experience shame and fear but the other person is in "level one" and longing for passion, excitement and uncomplicated high energy sex. If there are other unresolved issues between partners, this disharmony in their sexuality can easily become a central focus of conflict. One client told us that her boyfriend blamed their sexual problems on the workshops she was doing because, he said, "it has made everything difficult. Before you started going to all those seminars, our sex was fine. Now, you can't even open and enjoy yourself anymore."

For two people to be able to handle this difference, the love between them needs to be strong enough to allow them to work through it and to understand what is happening. Furthermore, in our experience, in some mysterious way, in a deep relationship people often mirror each other's state of fear or shame. It usually shows itself in different ways. One person may be more successful in his or her compensations, but deep down the wounds are often equal in strength. A problem arises if one partner is not willing to look at him or herself more deeply and how the relationship can be mirroring something that he or she is not yet in touch with.

The key for healing when you find yourself in "level two" is to begin to understand and validate your insecurity and fear. It also includes learning to give to yourself what you need to feel safe and open. When fear or insecurity is showing itself in your sexuality, you need tremendous patience and acceptance for the fear, shame and shock that is inside your body and your nervous system. That patience and understanding begins with being gentle with yourself and communicating with your partner.

Intimacy can only grow and deepen when we learn to validate each other's vulnerability. And then, strangely enough, our sexuality gets better as well.

"Level Three Sex"

"Level three sex" embraces whatever comes. Love becomes a container that holds the fear and the insecurity that may come up in your sexuality. When you have the feeling that you love your partner so much that you are patient and understanding for his or her fears, you are in "level three." When you have the feeling that you can be patient with your own fears and you know that you are loved with or without them, you are in "level three."

At this level, you are able to include, embrace, and even celebrate whatever arises when you are making love. This level is a true flowering of your essential nature of love — both for yourself and for another. There is acceptance of your vulnerability and this acceptance allows you to open sexually. In "level three sex," you accept what is happening. At this level, both you and your partner have arrived at the understanding that it is the love that matters, not the sexual high.

> *In" level three sex," the priority in sex is love and connection rather than sexual satisfaction. When we can begin to accept and even share our sexual fears and insecurities, self-trust and mutual trust grows.*

And as trust grows and you validate your vulnerability, it is much easier to express what you need. This acceptance and willingness to share in turn builds deeper trust. And paradoxically, as trust and love grows, often there is more space to include the passion and intensity that may have been frightening before. One woman shared with us that when she was able to validate and share with her husband the fears that came up for her while making love, and feel listened to and taken in by him, she was able to enjoy passion and orgasm in a way that she never had before. At this point, orgasm and excitement can happen or not, the sexuality can be more still and non-active, dysfunction can happen or not, it doesn't matter.

> *In "level three sex", we are naturally concerned with making it safe for our partner.*

With trust it becomes easier, even inviting, to share such delicate and sensitive things with each other because it only deepens the intimacy. Also, when love and intimacy is deep, you start to see that you can learn from each other's experience.

You are basically not so different from your partner. You can relate to your beloved's fears and insecurities because you also have them, even if they show differently. You no longer see a division. In fact, feeling and taking in the other person's vulnerability is one of the main ways that you can grow.

One couple shared with us that when they learned about how vulnerability affects sexuality, it changed their perspective. Rather than focusing on "getting off," they both became more receptive to each other's fears and could feel how this sensitivity was only making their love for each other deeper and richer.

At "level three," sex may naturally become more of a spiritual rather than a physical experience. Lovemaking becomes not only an experience of sharing love but also an experience of meditation. When there is a foundation of love, the two bodies and energies begin to melt. Rather than making love for release, you are making love for deepening of connection, presence and inner stillness. Excitement may fade with intimacy but it gets replaced by becoming deeply nourished with the connection, stillness and presence.

What we call "level three sex" is not only the flowering of love but also the flowering of a deeper self-awareness and understanding. It is the result of a journey we will describe in the chapters that follow. A journey of:

- Learning to love your body and celebrate your sexuality;
- Recognizing when you are using sex as a way of distracting yourself from feeling and being present to your vulnerabilities;
- Learning to honor your sexual needs, your own tempo and to validate your fears and insecurities;
- Learning to work through the emotional conflicts of intimacy that can affect your desire to make love and your experience of making love;
- Learning to listen to what you need moment to moment;
- Learning to respect and take in the other person's tempo, fears and insecurities;
- Taking care to create the time to make love away from the tensions of life and the pull of practical details that can easily swamp you and distract you from making love;

- Becoming aware that lovemaking can actually be a spiritual path that can nourish your deepest spiritual thirst by teaching you what love and meditation is.

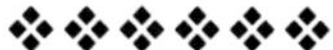

Part II

The Ways Sexuality Breaks Down

Chapter 2
"Am I Living My Sexuality?" The Longing For Sexual Freedom

Recently, in one of our training sessions, while working with sexuality, one of the men shared with the group, "I want to expose that I watch porn films and I'm not sure how to deal with this behavior. I feel guilty about it but I do it anyway."

He wanted our reaction as group leaders and feedback from the other group participants. The reaction from the group was mixed. Some of the women did not feel comfortable that he was doing this and wanted to know why he felt he needed to. He responded that he enjoyed the stimulation and it was a relief not to have to be concerned with all the "emotional stuff" that came up when he was making love with a woman. The reaction from the men was varied. Some admitted that they did it as well, others said that it was empty for them and that they would much rather make love in a way that was sensitive and loving.

We said, "In our view, watching pornography is not bad or wrong in itself. But it may be a symptom that something is missing in your life. There is a deep fear of intimacy or exposing fears and insecurities in lovemaking. Porn can become a way of your becoming sexually aroused without having to contend with another person. Watching pornography can turn on the body even though there is no current of love flowing between you and another person. In this way sex may become objectified and you are basically having sex with yourself — or rather, having sex with your mind."

"However, for you to choose not to watch porn just because you feel guilty and dirty doing it is not the answer. The answer is to bring your sexuality out of the shroud of guilt. Take a good look at all the judgments you have about being sexual, and to look at the negative messages about sex (both verbal and nonverbal) that you're are still carrying from your past conditioning. And does all that interfere with you learning to appreciate your body and your sexuality?"

"Tell you what," we added, "Describe to the group what you feel is true and authentic about your sexuality right now in your life."

"I love sex, I love to make love, and I love to make passionate love. I have a lot of shame about saying that, and I feel shame that sometimes I just want to make love even if I am not in love with the woman. But if I'm honest, that's what I feel. I was always taught that sex was something that one should hide and that just to feel sexual was not okay. Now, I want to live my sexuality, I want to explore my sexuality without always worrying about if I am in love or if the relationship is going somewhere."

When he shared this, he felt more relaxed and more accepting of himself. The women also said that they felt more comfortable with him now that he had been honest and open in this way. He was surprised to hear that some of them also liked to make love without being in love or without envisioning a long-term relationship with the sexual partner. On a deeper level, it would also be important for him, at some point, to explore his fears of coming closer to a woman. But this did not seem to be the time for this exploration. For now, he wanted (and needed) to bring his sexuality alive.

Sexuality is at the root of our life energy and when it is repressed, it creates an imbalance in our life energy as a whole. It can cause all kinds of physical and mental disturbances. Regardless of how much repression we may have been subjected to, the energy is so strong that it surfaces sooner or later. Sometimes it surfaces early and we begin as a teenager to explore our sexuality. But sometimes, we may have spent much of our adult life, even in a relationship, in sexual slumber.

A man shared with us that he married when he was in his early twenties. It was his first relationship as well as his first sexual experience with a woman. They were together for thirty years and then separated. During that time, he had fantasized about making love to other women but remained faithful to his wife. When the relationship ended, he went wild. His sexually alive teenager, which he had never lived, went on a rampage and he spent two years making love to many women, sometimes only for one night. Then he had enough. But he was happy that he had finally lived it out. Now he was together with a woman for two years, their sexuality was alive and healthy and he was no longer fantasizing about other women.

Many of us have received negative messages concerning sex, some of which may have come from our religious conditioning. Archaic messages such as:

- Sex is dirty, sinful or only for procreation;
- Sex is not spiritual or will distract you from God;
- Sex is unevolved and animalistic;
- Women should not desire sex, be active sexually, or initiate sex;
- Only have sex when you are married;
- Oral sex is perverted;
- It is not okay to be turned on by other men or women when you are in a relationship with someone;
- It is not okay to have sexual fantasies.

These messages are powerful and carry the weight of centuries of repression and guilt around sex.

We all got different sexual conditioning, but one thing is certain. If you have been raised in an environment in which sex was shrouded in guilt and repression and you took in these negative thought forms, you may judge your sexual energy and suffer from a constant state of guilt. These negative messages may not have come from your family but from the society you were raised in. You may find yourself in a deep split in which one part of you is attempting to be moral and righteous or spiritual and another part of you wants to play out your sexual desires with abandon. This split can easily begin to show itself in many ways, some of which are unhealthy. Rather than celebrating your sexuality, with full pleasure, fun and playfulness, you hide it. Rather than use sex as a playful adventure and a way of coming close to another person, you turn the other person into a sexual object. You split off our sex from your heart.

When we encounter people in our work who are living in a relationship where the sex has died, it can be because they may have ignored this situation because other factors in their lives took priority. But then often one of them meets someone new; falls in love, and the passion awakens. A couple in their late fifties had been married for thirty years and had two grown children. They came to work with us in separate workshops because their relationship was in trouble. Both were highly successful professionals. Two years previously, the man had fallen in love with a colleague and they had been having a passionate, clandestine love affair. Finally, he could no longer handle the deceit and told his wife of the affair. She was devastated, and he felt horribly guilty. His children were angry with him and blamed him for destroying the family. He and his wife attended a sexuality workshop to try to revive their sex life but he finally admitted that he was in love with this new woman and wanted to leave his wife.

There is always a possibility that the person who chooses to leave may be doing so because he or she does not want to deal with the emotional problems in the relationship and uses the affair as an escape. But it is also true that if you have repressed your sexuality and life presents you with a chance to live it out, the force of this energy is *very* strong. In this example, for the first time in this man's life, his sexuality was finally coming alive. He and his new lover came together to attend another one of our workshops and they were like two teenagers in love. He told us, with a somewhat sheepish smile, that they were making love three or four times a day and that he was making up for lost time, having sex in all kinds of strange, forbidden and exciting places — on airplanes in the bathroom, in the kitchen, on the living room floor. As time went on, their love deepened and they began to go through the levels that we described in the previous chapter.

It took some painful months for his wife to move through the grief of their separation but she had the courage to feel the pain and move through it. She is now enjoying her life in a new way, discovering what it means for her to be a woman living alone at this stage in her life. She began taking dance classes and applying to online dating programs to meet men.

The Danger of Spiritual Ideas

A man in workshop shared with us that he had been to a prostitute and withheld this secret from his wife. When she found out, she was upset, not so much that he had this adventure, but that he had not told her. He also told us that they had been practicing the technique of avoiding excitement and not having orgasm for some years and this was basically the only way that they made love these days. When we explored more deeply, he told us that he felt judged by her for still wanting to have passionate and hot sex sometimes and for having orgasms. He also judged what he called, "his sexual wild man." He is a well-known physician in his community and feels that it is not "right" for someone like him and of his age (50), to still have so such sexual energy and passion.

> *We can also repress our sexuality with spiritual ideas about what is "higher and more evolved." But often, our ideas come from an idea of where and who we should be rather than what is. Even when we learn new lovemaking techniques, this can also become just another form of repression — another morality, a new sexual religion.*

We guided him to feel and see the beauty, intensity and aliveness of his "sexual wild man." He could easily recognize that this was a wonderful side of him and admitted that although he liked their new way of making love, sometimes, he also liked to have hot sex, to be totally passionate and to have orgasms. We suggested that he share this openly with his partner.

The Pull To Be Alive vs. The Fear of the Unknown

Many people come together or even get married without having lived or explored their sexuality because their romance and relationship was an extension of their childhood conditioning. Also, in the hunger to find companionship, they may find themselves fixed into a long-term relationship long before they were ready. People can get married at a young age because conformity and security still commands their decisions. But there is also a force inside which wants to break out of the old, the stale and the known. Then you may find yourself torn between wanting to be alive but fearing the chaos that it can bring, between wanting to explore your sexuality and not wanting to upset the comfort and security of your life.

If you have spent years denying your life energy — and, more specifically, your sexual energy — and have put your energy and focus elsewhere, it can be disruptive to open up this box. It could mean disturbing the harmony and routine that you have created in your life, especially if you are in a relationship. But at some point, the longing for sexual freedom can motivate you to discover that something is missing.

Recently, we did a session with a woman in her early sixties who had fallen desperately in love with a man and was carrying on an affair even though she was still married and living with her husband of thirty-five years. She admitted that she was bored with her husband, that their life together had descended into tedious routines and that there was no real communication between them. She married him because he was such a stable man, financially secure, a warm-hearted person, and a loving father. Sex had ended years ago and she never really enjoyed it in the first place. But now, with this new man, she was exploding.

She felt like a horny teenager and was embarrassed lest her children find out. She had been honest with her husband about the situation, but divorcing him and disrupting the family seemed unthinkable. She came to us because she felt so confused, disturbed and seemingly out of control. We supported her to continue with this new man and pointed out that it was a healthy sign that she was waking up the life energy that she had repressed so many years ago.

It is important not to underestimate the power of these two conflicting forces — the desire for aliveness and the fear, even terror, of the unknown. The woman from the example above could not find the courage to leave her husband. We saw her at regular intervals for several years when she would come back either for a session or simply call to say hello. She was still attempting to juggle both men, and feeling horribly guilty toward both for not being able to make up her mind. Her excuse was that her children would never forgive her even though they were both fully grown and on their own. We simply supported her to keep feeling both sides of her conflict and allow time to work it out one way or another.

Every situation is different. But sometimes, it takes an affair to awaken you to the fact that you are denying your life energy and your sexuality. Sometimes it can motivate you to realize that the relationship you are in no longer works for you and it is time to move on.

Learning To Openly Communicate About Sex

One thing that helps awaken your sexuality is to start learning how to communicate about sex and to overcome some of your inhibitions of talking about it. We have an exercise in one of our workshops in which people are invited to share with their partner how they enjoy to make love - what makes them feel pleasure, what allows them to feel open and safe, what they like and don't like and what insecurities and shame they may have about sex. While it is easier to do this within the structure and safety of a group setting, it is also possible to do this kind of sharing with your lover when you are alone.

It is a challenge for a couple whose sex has diminished or died to resuscitate it but we have experience with couples who are ready to do whatever it takes to awaken their sexuality.

> *When we open the door to truth and aliveness, anything is possible. We just have to be willing to go with whatever life brings. Sometimes it means that the relationship will end and sometimes it means that intimacy and nourishing sex is just getting started.*

One example comes to mind of a couple that was able to make the transition out of sexual repression and to use this adventure to deepen their love for each other. We noticed, in the first group they did with us, that they behaved very strangely with each other. She was flirting with other men and he was becoming more and more withdrawn and silent. When we brought it up in the group, she admitted that she was attracted to another person and that she no longer felt sexually attracted to her husband. She complained that he was not a challenge for her, that he was not free sexually, was always trying to rescue her, and she felt bored. They were still in their twenties but had been married for several years. Neither of them had had any previous lovers; they were childhood sweethearts and married soon after graduating from high school.

Now, she was feeling the desire to make love to other men. After she had shared, he admitted that he also was attracted to other women. In fact, he had been actively been flirting with someone and had almost made love with her. Although hearing each other express themselves so honestly was shocking and painful, they said it was a relief at least to admit to themselves what was happening and finally to be honest about it with each other.

They continued to do workshops to learn more about themselves and learned to make love in a way that could help them develop their closeness. When we last heard from them, they were doing well. Their love for each other was strong enough to make the transition to intimacy. They no longer felt drawn to making love to others and were exploring being with each other in new and deeper ways.

Living Out Passion Creates Space for Deepening

When I (Amana) was in my early twenties I met a man, eleven years my senior, who woke me up sexually. With him my whole body came alive. I also had never experienced passion and desire like that before. I had been with many partners in my teenage years, exploring and enjoying being desired by men, but I had never felt this fire and passion myself. When I first met him he was still in a long-term relationship with a woman. We spent a passionate week together but I didn't think I would see him again because he was returning to his home, and to his relationship that was in a city a long way from mine.

However, to my great surprise, he told his partner about our affair, broke their relationship, and we moved in together. This was the beginning of a new life for me — a life of color, passion and love. This passion eventually opened a deep longing for a connection with something higher; it awoke our spirituality and we began searching for ways to connect deeper. We stayed together for five years but our lifestyles were too different. He wanted children and I didn't, and eventually we discovered that we needed to go separate ways.

In our experience, both in our own lives and also with other couples who have been together for a long time, if you allow yourself to live your passion out totally, after a while, you may want something else. You may begin to long for more closeness, connection, silence, and more depth in your lovemaking. And this passion may even wake up a deeper longing to know yourself and to reach the source of life. However, if you have not enjoyed hot, passionate sex, your attempts to bypass this phase and move directly into more meditative lovemaking may be just a spiritual idea and not your reality.

If you learn to trust your body and your sexual energy as it shows itself each moment, you may also discover that you long for something different than just passionate and orgasmic sex. And you may discover that sometimes you want to have hot, passionate sex but other times, you would prefer to move into softer, more meditative sex. Without the idea that one is better, higher, more spiritual, more alive, more real than the other, you can flow with whatever is there. However, excitement, as we will talk about in the next chapter, can be a form of addiction. And it naturally declines as intimacy deepens. What replaces excitement, however, is a much more nourishing flow of love, connection and depth.

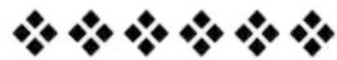

Chapter 3
"What Am I Running Away From?" Using Sex to Avoid Vulnerability

A former client and now friend of ours told us an interesting story. He is a world-class athlete and well known in his home country. For years, he used his fame to seduce women and have short-term, passionate sexual relationships with them. These relationships would last a year at the most and then he would move on to greener pastures. In-between women, he masturbated to relieve tension. In spite of his fame, his excellence in his sport and the constant availability of new attractive women, he felt emptiness in his life. Years ago, he began working intensively with himself in individual and group therapy. Still, nothing much changed in his relating patterns.

Then a close friend confronted him with the fact that he was a "sex addict" and told him that no matter how much therapy he did, no matter how deeply he delved into his childhood wounds, nothing would change until he stopped his addiction. At that moment, something clicked inside. He knew she was telling him the truth. He knew that what he had long considered being "sexual liberated" was just a mask for an addiction that was out of control. He joined Sex and Love Addicts Anonymous and began working a twelve-step program. At the time he shared this with us, he was working the fourth step - writing a moral inventory. He has stopped masturbating; he has stopped picking up women, and does not have sex with those he meets. He tells us that if he starts a new relationship with a woman, he will continue seeing her only if he sees the possibility of a long-term relationship and he will wait three months before making love. (Actually, the last time I spoke to him, he had been several months with a woman and felt that he finally was ready to be committed and monogamous.)

"You know, " he told us, "I did a workshop with you two ten years ago and at that time, I didn't have a clue that I was a sex addict and neither did you."

"Honestly," we told him, "at that time, we didn't even know what sex addiction was."

"I have to tell you," he added, "that something in your approach was missing. You could take us deep into our wounds and teach us to feel, understand and accept them, but you never really addressed addictive behavior. I am convinced now that just dealing with the wounds, even feeling them, isn't enough. I had to stop acting out from my addiction. When I started to do that, I began to contact fears and depths of loneliness and neediness that I never even imagined I had."

Our talks with him affected us deeply for many reasons. First of all, neither of us was informed about the prevalence and the importance of addressing the phenomenon of sexual addiction. My personal (Krish) orientation had been much more focused in helping myself and people I worked with to overcome sexual repression. Also, being the highly disciplined person that I am, addiction was not really one of my issues unless I considered discipline to be an addiction (which it has been for me). But neither of us has had to grapple with the difficulties of being enslaved by a behavior or a substance. Yet, increasingly, we have come to see that sexual behaviors that sabotage intimacy are a major factor in relationship dysfunction.

It has helped us to modify our approach. Now, we address the behavior directly as well as working with the underlying roots of dysfunction, whatever they are. And specifically, what we have learned about sex addiction both from our talks with him and our own study and experience, has opened our eyes. It is a much more common phenomenon that we realized.

Liberation or Addiction?

A couple came to see us who were having trouble because the man wanted to make love to other women and had told his partner that he actually did make love with another woman some weeks ago. The couple had only been together for a few months, and even though he enjoyed being with her he was convinced that it was necessary for his growth and his freedom to have multiple partners. The woman felt deeply threatened by this and said that she could not see how she could continue unless he changed his attitude.

To fully understand the situation we needed to know if he was interested in a deep and intimate relationship or if his priority was to explore sexually with different partners. We needed to know if, because of a past history of sexual repression and not living out his sexuality, he wanted, and even needed, to experiment sexually and it was not the time for him to enter into a more committed relationship. Or was he using this behavior as a way of avoiding depth and intimacy? This is an important question to ask ourselves if we are in a similar situation.

The man in this example came from a background with a strong and domineering mother. He admitted that whenever he came close to a woman, it brought up such terrible fears of losing himself and being swallowed by the woman that he felt he had to find some way to preserve his "manhood." The way he had habitually chosen to do this was to find other sexual partners. He could not see that he was using sex as a way of not feeling his fear. He was convinced that having multiple sexual partners was his freedom and that being in an "open relationship" was a more evolved way of being. The woman stood her ground and said that she could not tolerate being in a relationship with this kind of arrangement.

At the end of our session, things between them were not resolved. He was not convinced that it was the right thing for him to stop seeing other women. He still insisted that it was a compromise and a bourgeois way of living to settle down with one person. Eventually, they split up because the woman realized that it was only re-enforcing her shame to be in this kind of a relationship. She realized that she deserved to be with a man for whom she was enough. And she also realized that her "ex" was a sex addict. Sometimes the craving for "sexual liberation" can be a subtle mask for unacknowledged sex addiction.

> *Sex becomes an addiction when we use it to avoid feeling our fears and insecurities. Profound fear, shame and shock is a layer of our being which we have to explore if we want to know and accept ourselves deeply. But often it takes the longing for deeper intimacy to help us overcome sexual addiction.*

"Objective Sex" or "Subjective Sex"

A client of ours complained that her husband was secretly watching pornography on the Internet, and this brought up a lot of shame for her. It also caused her to distance herself from him sexually. When she confronted him with this behavior, he was overcome with guilt and promised to stop. But to her dismay, the behavior didn't stop and he would take opportunities when she was out of the house to go surfing online. When we worked with him on this issue, he could not understand what the attraction was but admitted that it was a way of feeling stimulated without feeling the usual fear that comes up when he gets close to his wife — or any woman for that matter. He had been sexually traumatized by the inappropriate and intrusive behavior of his mother, and opening sexually has always been a threatening challenge for him.

The attraction to pornography is HUGE. When this issue comes up in our workshops and we have asked people how many watch porn, many of the men have raised their hands and so have some of the women. Watching pornography can be a sign that we have not been taught a healthy approach toward sex since childhood and lacked an opportunity to explore our sexuality. Now, there is a hunger for such experiences. People and even some couples may watch pornography to jumpstart their sexuality — using it to stimulate their sexuality because of inhibitions that have developed inside.

Or, they use it because they have gotten lost in the practical and stressful aspects of every day life. But sex at this level can encourage fantasy rather than staying present while making love. The danger of watching pornography to get turned on is that it can easily become an addiction — an easy rush — but one that can prevent deeper connection with a partner and also prevents a deeper connection with yourself.

In another case, a man shared that he was most turned on with his wife when he fantasized about being dominated by women while making love. However, the attraction and excitement diminished when the lovemaking involved staying connected with her. His wife tolerated this behavior because she knew that it was pleasurable for him, but it disturbed her because she felt objectified. He also had been sexually traumatized when he was a child by his mother, who would invite him into her bed and allow him to rub up against her.

Pornography, objectifying fantasies, or having frequent and varied sexual partners, can be a sign of sexual addiction. You don't have to face the complex emotional issues that come up when you come closer to someone. It can allow stimulation and excitement without having to go into the fears and insecurities that commonly arise when you come closer to someone. It can be very important to have "objective sex" in order to revive and explore sexual energy and to overcome old inhibitions and judgments.

> *Uncomplicated sex is very fulfilling on one level because you may not be so disturbed by your insecurities and fears. You may be able to function more effectively and experience more pleasure and excitement than when you become intimate with someone and begin to touch insecurities.*

But "objective sex" not only has nothing to do with intimacy, it can damage the closeness, trust and connection that we have with someone. It may be exciting when you use fantasies, pornography or sex games, but it begins to take a toll. You can build a wall between yourself and the other person. You are going against the natural flow of life. As you come closer to someone, deeper levels will open. When you try to keep the sex objective, you are hiding these deeper levels from your partner — and perhaps from yourself as well.

Instead, if you keep a continual connection to your partner while making love, the sexuality becomes subjective. "Subjective sex" offers the reward to tremendous nourishment, but along the way you may have to encounter fears and insecurities that you have avoided. It is a rite of passage. It takes tremendous trust for two people to open to each other.

> *Once we start to allow ourselves to become vulnerable, we're going to touch our deepest fears. That is what intimacy means. As the trust grows and as these deep fears start to come up, running off to have sex with another person or escaping into fantasies or porn can easily be running from our own vulnerability — in short, sexual addiction.*

The initial excitement and high energy that was there may begin to be replaced by fears, and the body may start to show this fear in many ways. This is uncomfortable, especially if you have no idea what is happening or why, and don't welcome this different level of sexuality. When this starts to happen, you can easily feel drawn to making love with a stranger where you can function again as you did before and feel the heat and excitement again. Or you may become frustrated with your partner's fears and want to have sex with someone whose sexuality is not being affected by fear or insecurity.

Anne was married with two children but began having affairs. She defended this behavior because she felt it was her need to be free and alive and she felt too confined in the relationship with her husband. The sex was no longer what it used to be and she was missing "good sex." Eventually, her husband had had enough and they got a divorce. However, she still felt drawn to her husband and found herself spending vacations with him. They were not lovers, but she noticed that she was beginning to feel attracted to him again. She had had other lovers, but somehow she kept coming back to her connection with her ex-husband.

It took a few workshops before she began to touch what was underneath. Anne had no trouble with sexual repression and inhibitions. She had been sexually active since her early teens and described herself as wild and adventurous when it came to sex. But when she became vulnerable with a man, she began to feel such profound fear that her body would freeze and her sexual desire would vanish. After some exploration through the body, she began to connect with sensations and even memories of being sexually abused. She recognized that she was terrified to open her body deeply to a man and to becoming vulnerable. Now she could see that her affairs were a way of not feeling this terror.

Excitement or Addiction?

We would like to stress that even though it is important to awaken your repressed sexuality, it is also important to realize that sex and love are not the same. When you come out of repression or when you meet someone who awakens your sexuality in a way that you have never experienced before, it is like a drug. It is a wonderful drug, but one that is often mistaken for love. This misunderstanding can create much confusion because when people enter into a powerful and nourishing sexual connection, it opens up energy that they may have repressed and they think they are in love.

The heart may open and they may feel powerfully expanded. But it isn't love. Love is a challenging process of learning to be sensitive, loving and respectful of yourself and your partner. It is something that requires self-awareness and self-love combined with the understanding that to live in harmony with another human being you need to develop profound trust and respect for each other as well as for yourself.

A couple in one of our workshops shared that they were fighting much of the time and their sex life was dead. When we asked them questions about their relationship, we learned that they had come together because the sex "was so great." The man admitted that when he met his wife, he felt lonely and the sexual attraction was very strong. It was the best sex he had ever had and he couldn't get enough. He wanted to make love all the time. He even wanted to have a child together (which they did). Then everything changed. She felt he was not living up to his responsibilities to help take care of the child and he became resentful, more demanding and less sensitive in their sex. They lost the attraction for each other, moved to separate bedrooms and quarreled. They tried to build a relationship on sex alone and it failed.

It is possible to build intimacy where there had only been a sexual connection but you have to work through many stages of good times and hard times. Hostility, disappointment and resentment naturally build up in most long-term relationships and you need to learn the tools for how to work through the difficult times.

I (Krish) had several experiences in my life where I confused a powerful sexual connection for love. Some years ago, I met a woman who was in a relationship with another man and we secretly made dates to make love. Up until then, I had never been with someone who was so fulfilling sexually. I was convinced that I was totally in love and that what we had was much more than sex. After one of our nights together, I longed for our next encounter and suffered in-between. But from the beginning, she told me that while we obviously shared something special and beautiful, we were not meant to be in a longer relationship. I didn't believe her until much later. Finally, our meetings became too disruptive for her relationship and she cut it off.

As we mentioned in the introduction, many years ago, when Amana and I began our relationship, we participated in a sexuality workshop that taught lovemaking without excitement and orgasm. In the course of the workshop, I realized how addicted I was to the excitement of sex and that the feeling of excitement was very tied to anticipating and having an orgasm (and also my partner having an orgasm.) By learning to make love without coming, it caused a shift in my awareness.

I noticed that when I was no longer focused on excitement and anticipating orgasm, I was able to be more present to what was happening in my body, to Amana and to our connection together. And the quality of the lovemaking changed. It became longer, slower and more still. Most of the time now, we make love in this way. Sometimes we make love with excitement and orgasm and totally enjoy it. But before I learned to make love this way, I never could have imagined that there was another way to make love and that sex could be fulfilling without the excitement and the anticipation of orgasm.

> *Because the sexual energy is so intense and so compelling, it can become obsessive. This addiction to excitement naturally can cause us also to be focused on performance and maximizing pleasure. Many people have the idea that "good sex" means having an orgasm, making sure that the partner has an orgasm, and even trying to ensure that both come at the same time. This idea of "good sex" creates tremendous pressure and it may easily leads us to become compensated when we are making love.*

When that occurs, you're no longer open to what is happening inside each moment because you have an agenda about what "should" happen. When you bring this kind of attitude to your lovemaking, anything that interferes with performance and pleasure is a disturbance. Then you may be reluctant to allow your vulnerability to surface as this could interfere or dampen the sexual fire.

The obsession with performance, excitement and hot sex not only can create stress but it can easily interfere with deep intimate connection. Ariel is a young, attractive and very alive man whose main preoccupation, for the first years that he worked with us, was how to find women to sleep with. He felt that he was sexually competent and complained that he had trouble finding women who were fully orgasmic and alive enough. He was frequently disappointed not only because women did not live up to his standards but also because women rejected him after a few dates and he could not understand why.

He complained to us, "Women are so repressed that they can't just enjoy sex for sex's sake. They are afraid of energy and are stuck on this idea of commitment. To me, it's just a way of avoiding life and wanting everything to be safe. Life's isn't about safety; it's about energy and aliveness. It's unpredictable. If you ask me, underneath it all, they simply want to control men."

Initially, when we suggested to him that his approach to sex was addictive and the way he was treating women was abusive, he was outraged. He could not see how being "juicy" and "alive" had anything to do with addiction or how wanting to have passionate, hot, uncommitted sex was abusive. But he also had a sincere willingness to grow, and in time he began to realize that there must be something in him that caused this reaction from women. He saw that the way he was relating to women and making love was disconnected. He was avoiding his vulnerability.

Slowly, he began to feel the depth of his insecurity and the fear that if he ever exposed his vulnerability he would be rejected, controlled or shamed. And as he became more conscious of this insecurity, he realized that he did not want to continue to repeat his old habits. He had the strength to stop trying to seduce women. Since he did not yet know another way to approach women, he stopped having sex.

This abstention felt to him as though he was going "cold turkey." He was used to having sex on a regular basis and without this continual form of release, it brought up a great deal of anxiety. For a while he masturbated to relieve the tension, but then he stopped doing that as well.

Having the understanding that he gained from working with himself, he could handle the anxiety and put his prodigious energy into his creativity. He began a clothing business and in a matter of two years, he was already well on his way to financial success. When he began to make love again, it came as a shock to him to realize how much he had used women in the past just to satisfy his need for release.

"I'd rather be alone," he told us, "than be driven by that energy. I don't need to be a slave to my addiction for sex. It's not easy and sometimes I don't know what to do with the tension that I feel inside, but it's worth it. I also can see why women pulled away from me. My approach was manipulative."

Because of his courage and willingness to go through this healing process, he was becoming a different person — more mature, more trustworthy and more respectful.

Sexual Acting Out

The levels of sexual addiction can be subtle. One of its more disguised forms is sexual acting out. Sexual seduction games whether in a man or in a woman are most often a cover for not wanting to feel your fears, insecurities and helplessness. Susanna is a sexy, alive and attractive Brazilian woman in her early thirties. The clothes she wears, while not particularly remarkable in Brazil, are unusually provocative anywhere else. It never occurred to her that there was anything unusual about the way she dressed, even though it had a pronounced affect on those around her.

But when she began to work sincerely and deeply with herself, bringing awareness to her wounds and to the ways that she compensated for them, she began to see that her dressing style was not totally innocent. She was using it to feel her power and to cover up her insecurities. What she took for natural, spontaneous aliveness and simply "strutting her stuff" was also a masquerade for fears and shame. Inside, she felt that without her beauty and sex appeal, she was nothing.

Sexual acting out often occurs when someone has a history of sexual abuse. One common result of sexual trauma is to become sexualized. A child who is abused by an adult learns that he or she gets love and attention by being seductive. From our experience, often when someone is using sex for attention, he or she has a history of sexual abuse in some form. What may seem as sexy and seductive is actual a cover for deep inner pain.

Beatrice came to a workshop with her boyfriend dressed very provocatively and flirting with many of the men even from the first session. We noticed her behavior and suspected that she might be covering up a history of sexual abuse. On the third day, in a structure in which we invited people to form a sculpture of their traumatized child using a partner as their model, she exposed her abuse story to the group.

You can also extend your sexually acting-out behavior to the ways in which you make love. A couple we worked with years ago told us that they liked to make love with bondage. They took turns tying each other up and having sex in this way. At the time, they were both convinced that this was a perfectly acceptable way of making love. It was exciting and adventurous and they had no intention of letting go of it or even considering that it might be a compensation for something deeper. Later, the woman discovered that she was a survivor of severe sexual abuse.

Once having uncovered and worked with this wound, she found she could no longer make love in this way. When you have been abused sexually or physically, you can easily act out your trauma in sex either as a victim or as a perpetrator. Often, when you have experienced a sexual trauma, you are disconnected from your body while making love because of your fear. You may be drawn to sexual acting out in lovemaking, to games and sex toys, even drawn to having hard or painful sex just to feel something.

There is no formula for determining whether sex is just exploration or it has become an addiction. Sexual exploration can be the right thing for someone who has repressed his or her sexuality and wants to break free from this life-negative conditioning. But when you are habitually using sex to avoid closeness or to avoid feeling your shame, pain and fear, it is different. Then it has become an addiction that can keep you from facing yourself or from becoming intimate with another person.

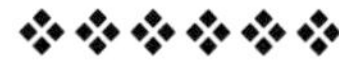

Chapter 4
"Why Don't I Feel Anything?" How Shock Affects Our Sexuality

We're now going to be exploring more deeply what happens in "level two sex." It's our experience that in most long-term relationships, issues come up which create disturbance in sexuality. This can happen for both people but often it is one person who first begins to encounter difficulties. We find that these difficulties come in three ways. The first is fear. It can show itself as a body dysfunction, as no longer being present while making love or as not wanting to make love.

The second is shame. Shame can cause us to compromise or compensate in our lovemaking or can also cause us to pull away, isolate and become depressed or resigned.

And the third is a growing mistrust of our partner. This mistrust can arise because we don't feel that the person is attentive to our needs and sensitivities or we don't feel met energetically. In this chapter we will focus on fear, looking at how fear, shock and dysfunction affects our sexuality.

A woman in one of our yearlong trainings was sharing that when she began making love in a slower way, with focus on feeling her body instead of the usual program of excitement and orgasm, at first it was sheer delight. She felt a much deeper and more heartfelt connection to her boyfriend and they could make love for a long time. But as the lovemaking went deeper, she began to reach a point where she went numb.

"I couldn't feel anything," she said, "and that frustrated me and made me want to return to the old way where at least I could feel something. Now learning about shock, it gives me a framework to understand what this feeling of numbness is and helps me understand that there is nothing wrong with me."

Shock and Dysfunction are Hidden Symptoms of Fear

When you open deeper places in your being, your sexuality may need to adjust to this change. It is natural and predictable that as familiarity, safety and trust grows, you become more vulnerable, particularly when you are making love. This change may not happen for both people in a relationship in the same way or at the same time. But if the love is deep and there is a willingness to learn, grow and allow change, your sexuality can adapt and intimacy deepen. For this to happen, you need to understand that as vulnerability opens, so do many unconscious fears.

Fear shows itself in the most familiar way as panic, nervousness, agitation, shaking, sweating, rapid heartbeat and restlessness. When you notice these symptoms it is easier to recognize that you have fear. However, fear may also present itself as an absence of feeling or as a dysfunction. You may notice that you are not feeling your body or your emotions or that something is not working the way you would like it to. Sexual dysfunctions are very common.

Most of us would prefer that they disappear without the slightest interest in exploring where they come from. Trouble is, they don't just go away. Any kind of pressure you may put on yourself to feel anything or for the body to work in the way you would like it to, only makes them worse. Dysfunctions come from profound shock. When there is pressure, the shock gets worse and so do the dysfunctions.

A woman was sharing with us that she had begun a new relationship with a man who was a colleague at work. After being friends for a long time, they both realized that the attraction for each other was very strong.

Yet they both hesitated to move into sex because he was married and had a child. But finally they decided to spend the night together. He said that he no longer loved his wife and felt that the relationship with her was over. Still, the idea of betraying her and the child by making love to another woman brought up tremendous guilt. In their lovemaking, he lost his erection and felt horribly ashamed. She was loving and aware enough to explain to him that it was natural reaction to his guilt and fear of betraying his family.

Fear, shock and dysfunction are closely related. Shock is frozen fear. A dysfunction is a symptom of fear lodged in the body and nervous system and expressed as something not working in the body. Sexual dysfunctions may have a physical component but most often they are shock symptoms covering fear and/or guilt. Sometimes these sexual dysfunctions show themselves only after you have come closer to a person and sometimes they occur whenever you make love regardless for how long you have been with someone.

Before I (Krish) learned about shock, I didn't know that when I lost control of my ejaculation it was because of shock. Or that the shock was coming from deeply seated fear. Over time, I've explored the origin of this fear, but what has been most helpful for me is simply recognizing that dysfunction is shock and shock is fear.

What is most transformational is not necessarily knowing where our fear or shock comes from but knowing that it is fear and feeling and accepting it when it comes up.

It's helpful to understand what is behind a body dysfunction. When the body does not respond the way you would like it to, it is because you are feeling fear, pure and simple. But much of the time you're not in touch with this fear because it's deeply buried in your unconscious. A stimulus provokes a body memory of something having happened to you in the past that was terrifying. At the time that it occurred, you didn't have the resources to understand, defend or cope with the frightening experience.

You bury it in the subconscious. But the stimulus brings up the fear that you have stored in your nervous system. Now, in response to this trigger, you shut down or your body creates some kind of a symptom as a way of holding down the anxiety. That shutting down or pushing away is dysfunction.

What is Shock?

When you're in shock, often you can't move, feel, talk or think clearly. You're frozen, confused and terrified (even though you may not know it). The nervous system is built to respond to threat and invasion by either confronting the threat or fleeing from it — fight or flight. In the past when you have experienced countless insensitivities, invasions or even abuses, you lacked the ability to respond in either of these two ways – to run away or to confront the person or situation that was frightening you. I (Krish) studied with psychologist Peter Levine, Ph.D. et al, in a three-year trauma-healing training where I learning many of these concepts. [See his book, *Waking the Tiger* in the selected references.]

The third alternative, and the only one available to you at the time, was to freeze. This freezing includes shutting down your life energy and pulling inside where you can feel safe. Sometimes you pull the energy so deeply inside that you disconnect your attention and awareness from the outside even to the point of dissociating from your body. This is why when you are in shock, you often space out, become non-responsive or non-reactive and you don't hear, see or understand things on the outside clearly.

How Shock Shows in Your Life

Even though the traumas that caused the freezing may have happened long ago, your nervous system still holds the trauma inside. A slightest trigger can bring up the panic and the shock. In its more unconscious or hidden form, the shock can present as, for instance, skin diseases, asthma, disorders of the nervous system, lower back and disk problems, irritable bowel syndrome or colitis, as the feeling of having to urinate repeatedly, or as confusion and disorientation. When the fear comes more to the surface, it can show itself as hypervigilance, hyperactivity, phobias, panic attacks, perpetual anxiety, irritability, or outbursts of rage. Sometimes, shock shows itself as a general lowering of your life energy and particularly your sexual energy. If you have past trauma connected to being alive and expressive, you may find yourself not only avoiding sex but also dampening your life energy in all areas of life. Any increase in your expression of life energy becomes too frightening.

Ulrika is a sensitive and withdrawn woman in her early forties. She talks in a quiet and restrained voice and rarely shares in the open group. But when we put on dance music, she comes alive and it is as though she becomes a totally different person — full of life, sensuous and expressive. She tells us that in her daily life, she only feels alive and happy when she dances or plays her guitar. Mostly, she isolates herself in her apartment, watching television and going to bed, feeling depressed and lonely. In her childhood, she was not permitted to be alive and expressive. She remembers that when she did, she was punished. It has helped her to realize that she still carries this trauma inside. By taking small risks to meet people and express herself instead of isolating herself, she begins to experience that she won't get punished if she comes alive.

Gertrude is a young, attractive woman in her late twenties who speaks softly and appears introverted and self-contained. In her life, she has been strongly drawn to meditation, has spent many years living in meditation communities, and frequently goes to India to attend meditation retreats. When we got to know her better, we began to feel that she was hiding her sexuality and that her quiet demeanor was not only an expression of her essence, it was also a defense.

As she worked with us, her energy slowly began to come alive. She would go back and forth between expressing herself as a vibrant, powerful, sensuous woman and a terrified little girl. She began to realize that coming alive made her open to men's sexual attentions and it terrified her because her father was subtly sexual with her. By staying quiet, withdrawn and subdued, she was safe. Now her journey to heal this wound is to allow her aliveness and to learn to say "no" to men when something doesn't feel right to her.

How Your Shock Shows Itself in Your Sexuality

Sexuality is an area in which you're extremely vulnerable. For that reason, your shock is easily triggered in sex. When you have shock in connection to your sexuality, it doesn't necessary need to be coming from some past history of sexual trauma. It can be coming from any kind of trauma that you're still holding in your body from a prior trauma. When it shows in your sexuality, shock can present itself as a dysfunction, dissociating (going away), over-compensating while making love, a decrease in energy or interest in sex or becoming frozen and/or numb. When you dissociate, you're making love but you're not present. You are going through the motions but you're not really there.

> *When we're in shock we don't feel the body and therefore cannot feel when something isn't right for us. When we're in shock, it is extremely difficult to feel and express what we need, or to set a limit.*

I (Amana) remember many incidents as a teenager when I made love in a way that wasn't right for me. I allowed men to touch me in ways or participated in ways that did not feel right because I wasn't present and aware of how I felt about it. When you are in shock you may be so pulled inside that someone can make love to your body and even mistreat it, and you may feel as if they are not even touching you. The traumatic events that happened in the past caused you to find a safe place inside. But you may have no or little connection with other people and may feel as if your life is a movie in which you are simply a spectator.

Marianne and Phillip were having difficulties because she had lost all interest in sex. She did not know why at first, but after working with a therapist and later with us in several workshops, she discovered that she had experienced sexual abuse as a child from her father. For Phillip, it was a bewildering and difficult situation. He was a busy businessman who was not inclined toward therapy or working with childhood wounds. His life was functioning well, he was in love with his wife and his children and until this situation developed with Marianne, everything was going along perfectly well.

When they came to see us, she exposed her abuse story to him for the first time. Before, she had been too frightened and too ashamed to talk about it even with him. She expected him to discredit her story but, on the contrary, he wept and told her how sorry he felt for her and how enraged he felt toward her father. But their lack of sexuality was still a concern for him.

We explained that her aversion to sexuality was a natural result of her abuse.

"Yes," he asked, "but why didn't this come up sooner. Why now?"

"Because," we answered, "from our experience, often it happens this way. When we come closer to someone and trust grows, deeper places of past trauma begin to surface. And this is most common in our sexuality."

"Okay," he said, "but what do we do about it? I can't live without ever having sex."

"Marianne," we asked "is there was any way that you could imagine coming close to Phillip physically which would not be too overwhelming for you?"

"I think that we could hold each other but for now, I can't make love."

"How is that for you, Phillip?" we asked.

"I can live with that for awhile as long as it isn't forever."

We stayed in touch with them regularly over a three-year period. She came to more workshops and went through our yearlong training. She also continued to see her therapist weekly during the whole time. When we last saw them, they were doing well. He had come to accept her fear and the shock in her body and she had slowly been able to receive him sexually more often. It was a delicate process and not always smooth but for us, their story is an example that when the love is strong enough, it can transcend these difficulties.

Shock Triggers

Shock triggers are anything that makes you suspect that there is a threat. Often the trigger is not an actual threat but it is enough to cause your bodies to react and go into shock. Sometimes just a look from someone or the anticipation of something happening can be enough. It can come up, particularly in lovemaking, whenever you come closer to your partner, whenever you feel that he or she is not present or when you fear his or her angry. It can even come up when you sense any kind of pressure — even if it is unspoken. It can come up when you have to perform, when you feel tested, when you are in a new situation, when you try something new, or whenever you feel that the other person is insensitive with you. In fact, the more sensitive and vulnerable you feel, the easier it is for shock to come up.

Anita and Paul came to see us because of difficulties in their lovemaking. They had been together for five years and their difficulties only began a year ago.

Paul shared, "I feel upset because often when we are making love Anita suddenly pulls away. Sometimes we continue to make love but then I feel as though I am making love to someone who isn't there any longer. Other times, Anita just stops and tells me she can't continue. But she never says why she pulls away."

When we asked Anita to talk about how it was for her, she said, "I know that it is hard for him but I can't help it. When we start to make love, I am turned on and I want to make love and be close to Paul. But then something takes over in me and I don't even know what happens. It's as if I just can't be there anymore. I just want to be alone and I can't stand that Paul is so close. Sometimes I continue to make love because I feel so guilty and I don't want to hurt Paul. I know it's not fair, but I don't know what to do."

"Is there something that he does that frightens you?' we asked.

"To be honest," she said, "I have absolutely no idea. I don't even know if I am frightened. I just don't want to be there anymore."

"Has this happened to you before with other men in your past?" we asked.

"No, this is the first time anything like this has happened. But I've never loved anyone like I love Paul."

If you feel or project that someone is insensitive to you in lovemaking, not present, moving too fast, too demanding, aggressive and insensitive in any way, it can easily trigger you to go into shock and provoke dysfunction or other trauma symptoms. Your shock can be triggered if something makes you feel abandoned or even if you feel the fear of being abandoned while making love. Most of us are highly sensitive to rejection, and this sensitivity can be even stronger when it comes to sexuality. The sense that someone is not present or does not want to be with you or make love to you can be traumatic because it kindles your fears of abandonment. A related shock trigger can be feeling judged, criticized or even just anticipating judgment or criticism while making love.

But often you may not know what provokes your shock, and you may not even know that you are *in* shock. First of all, your shock can come up so quickly and so unexpectedly that it can take you totally by surprise. And, secondly, if you don't know about the phenomenon of shock and about the trauma that is underneath, you don't have a framework for receiving it. Until you understand about shock, it can seem like a terrible affliction, whenever you feel unable to function properly or whenever you feel frozen, disconnected or frightened while making love.

When shock or dysfunction shows itself in love making, we are no longer able to enjoy the innocent

> *and uncomplicated sex of "level one." When our vulnerability opens and our fears and insecurities start to show themselves, we are in "level two."*

If your only concern is to have hot, passionate sex, then you will fight with yourself and with your body because your vulnerability is interfering with how you want to make love. But, if you can welcome the fears that are showing themselves, even if you don't understand why they come or where they are coming from, they can become a doorway toward deeper love both with yourself and with your partner.

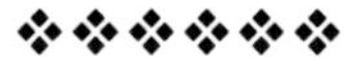

Chapter 5
"I Don't Deserve Anything Better." How Sex Brings Up Our Shame

Angela met a man at a party and began dating him. When they started to make love, she asked him to wear a condom. He did so reluctantly but while inserting the condom, it broke and he did not want to put on a new one, saying that he lost his sensitivity when he wore a condom. She complied, but later felt that she had betrayed herself.

Sonya was attracted to a man and was spending nights with him but without making love. She wanted to make love but he told her that he wasn't really interested in sex because he "didn't feel that way about her." She accepted this, hoping that eventually he would change his mind. In the meantime, she suffered. When we asked her why she put herself in this kind of situation, she admitted that she was used to being rejected by men and didn't expect to be desired.

These are two examples for how easily your insecurity can affect your sexuality. When you have lost touch with your self-worth, you feel that you don't deserve to be loved. This loss of self worth is called "shame." It is a deep feeling of insecurity and of not trusting or even knowing your feelings, an inner sense that you are fundamentally wrong, defective and inadequate. When you enter into relationships without knowing about and without having felt your shame, it deeply influences your relating and your sexuality. You may try to cover it or hide from it, but that does not make it go away. When you are in shame, you can oscillate between feeling worthless or feeling better than others, between collapse and grandiosity.

Nathan manifests his shame in its grandiose form. He teaches sexuality workshops and prides himself in his ability to be sensitive and present when making love. He is successful in his work, and his students admire his knowledge of sexuality and his skill at teaching tantric techniques. However, he has not been able to have intimacy with a woman. He has short affairs but invariably he "discovers" that the women he is with are not "deep, sensitive or present" enough for him, especially when they are making love. Underneath the mask of a proficient teacher is someone who is deeply insecure and lonely. But this part of him remains cloaked in denial. There is still too much fear for him to feel the shame.

Sometimes it takes an outside provocation — like a rejection, abandonment, judgment, criticism, failure, an accident or illness to help you realize that you have shame. When your shame is provoked, you may enter into deep self-doubt, depression and hopelessness, and may even have suicidal thoughts. And if you don't want to face and feel your shame, you can easily become angry, defensive, aggressive or self-destructive as an attempt to get away from the pain inside.

> *The experience of shame comes from a basic disconnection from ourselves — a state in which we are not in touch with our essential gifts and uniqueness and we're not resting in this knowing of ourselves. In this disconnected state, rather than feeling the divine presence that radiates through us in a unique and special way, we base our self-esteem on what others think about us, on our performance or on our image.*

There are few areas where image, performance and what others think of you hits you more strongly than in sex.

The Causes of Shame — in Sex and In Other Areas

Shame comes basically from not feeling seen and supported for who you are and who you can become. It can begin in infancy if you did not feel received or appreciated, or if there was tension and conflict in the environment in which you were raised. As a child, you assume responsibility for whatever unloving, unsupportive and even abusive energy you receive or feel around you. You develop a deeply negative self-image.

Tanya is an attractive, vivacious, highly intelligent petite woman in her mid-thirties. She was raised by a narcissistic and controlling mother and an absent father. As a teenager, she was rebellious and angry and was told, particularly by her mother that she was a difficult and negative person who created conflict wherever she was. Now, she continually blames herself whenever conflict arises with her family members or with men in her life, and is convinced that there is something basically dark and ugly about herself, that her heart is closed and that she incapable of love. Her negative self-image is a direct result of the abuse she received as a child and as an adolescent.

Although shaming is a general phenomenon that happens during childhood, there are some very specific factors which contribute to it:

- *Being unsupported or repressed in your natural life energy.* This includes your anger, sexuality, aliveness, joy, fear, and sadness. It can happen from direct verbal messages or simply from a negative attitude toward aliveness by those who raised you. Feeling and trusting your natural life energy is the first and most important way that you gain a positive sense of self. When this is unsupported or squashed, you lose a basic trust in yourself.
- *Being abused emotionally, physically or sexually by an adult, or even witnessing such abuse.* This creates profound guilt in a child, because his or her only way of making sense out of this kind of treatment is by assuming that he or she deserves it. Sexual abuse is even more confusing because a child may

enjoy the attention and the physical sensations but at the same time may feel horribly guilty and ashamed for enjoying it.

- *Being physically or emotionally abandoned as a child.* When you do not feel the presence, appreciation and embrace of a parent, you also imagine that you have done something wrong to make them go away.
- *Being raised by a narcissistic parent whose primary concern and energy was for her or himself.* With this kind of parenting, you miss the opportunity to be seen for who you are because you are always being seen as an extension to the parent's narcissistic needs. The mirroring of yourself that you receive has nothing to do with you and everything to do with the narcissistic parent.
- *Being patronized and cast into the role and image of a child.* Such treatment locks you into the experience of yourself as a child without the ability to grow up and stand on your own feet. This kind of shaming also includes parents who have an emotional (and unconscious) investment in keeping you a child to meet their own needs.
- *Being conditioned to play a role in the family or any kind of pressure and expectation to perform.* In some cases you gained approval for being a caretaker or a super-achiever, or in other cases you took on the opposite role of a clown or someone who fails in reaction to pressure or expectations. In fact, the pressure and expectations that may you may have received is deeply shaming because you come to believe that your worth depends on what you do rather than on who you are.
- *Being raised in an environment full of rules and regulations.* When a child's spontaneity and nature is restricted from an early age with rules and regulations, he or she never has a chance to explore. He or she begins to feel guilty about any

possible transgression and slowly adapts to becoming a good boy or girl. This can kill the fire of life.

- *Being infected by the negativity and fears of a caretaker.* A child naturally absorbs the energy and subtle vibrations of those taking care of him or her. He or she begins to believe what she feels and the negativity and fears of a parent become his or her own.
- *Being compared to someone.* A child who is compared either favorably or unfavorably to someone such as a sibling is shaming. The same is true when he or she feels pressured to perform up to a standard set by another.
- *Dishonesty and family secrets.* When a child is raised in an environment where there is dishonesty, it creates a profound feeling inside of unreality. He or she starts to doubt his or her own feelings and intuitions. This applies to factual as well as emotional dishonesty.
- *Being labeled or told what you are feeling and thinking.* A child who is labeled — told who he or she is or told what he or she is thinking or feeling is robbed of his or her essential trust of his or herself.
- *Being humiliated, teased, criticized or judged.* A child who has these experiences begins to form a deep self-image of shame. It may not seem damaging to the person handing out the attacks but it certainly does to a child.

The end result of any or all of this kind of shaming is that you grow up with a defective sense of self, believing all the negative, condemning voices that have become lodged in your mind. Perhaps you minimize and/or prematurely forgive your parents for these experiences before you have felt the injustice and the damage that they caused. Then you run the risk of keeping the shame for your whole life and allowing it to affect every aspect of your life.

Shame Leads Us to Compromise Sexually

Sara is a woman in her early fifties who came to us because her marriage of thirty years was in trouble. Her husband is a wealthy businessman who spends his time traveling the globe and has rarely been at home. She became used to waiting around for him and accepting what few crumbs of attention and lovemaking that he gave to her. In the course of the first workshop that she did with us, she learned from a friend, who was also attending, that her husband had been having affairs for years. She always suspected this, but it was devastating to have it confirmed and she felt humiliated that other people knew about it before her.

Sara's shame made her feel that she didn't deserve anything better. She compared herself endlessly with all the "young and attractive" women that he was sleeping with, and still could not imagine a life without him. She even admitted to us that although he was never really present or caring in their lovemaking, he was the one she was most attracted to sexually and could not imagine finding another man. Over a period of several years in which she attended many workshops with us, she slowly began to feel that she deserved more in her life. She awakened the rage she had inside for being so collapsed and compliant with him and for settling for so little.

From the reflections of other people in the workshops, particularly men, she began to recognize that she was someone people actually wanted to spend time with. It surprised her when many men told her that they found her attractive, feisty, funny, alive, sensitive and intelligent. Eventually, she got a divorce and began to experience life as a single woman. It is still new for her, but she is gradually beginning to come out of her shame and to feel her beauty, power and sensuality. She started an affair with someone that she had known for years and discovered that not all men made love with only their own needs in mind. Some men are caring and tender, and take the time to consider her and to pleasure her.

Because of shame, you give yourself away for love, you betray your body, you compromise your own needs, and you enter into situations in which you feel disrespected and even abused. Shame-based people are often more focused on pleasing or impressing the other person while making love than on staying true to themselves. Also, when you're shame-based, you may be more interested in proving to yourself or to your partner that you're performing well than in respecting yourself or having a deep and intimate connection with the other person. One client shared that he never feels himself when he is making love. His only concern is pleasing his lover. When she is pleased, he feels that he has done a good job and feels good about himself.

Shame Can Compel Us To Compensate in Sex

Shame not only causes you to compromise in sex, it also drives you to compensate in your lovemaking. The endless need to prove to yourself that you are "a good lover" and to cover the depth of your sexual insecurities is extremely common. In a couple's session we did recently, the woman claimed that when they made love, she could not feel her husband. She was angry because she felt that he was only interested in sex and not in connecting with her. He wanted to make love in "exciting" places and experiment with different positions, including anal sex. She appreciated his passion and his intensity but she felt that she was missing him.

I (Krish) have found (and I suspect it is true for many men) that the fear of not living up to my (or the other person's) expectations in sex had driven my lovemaking for a good percentage of my life. I was performing. Though I didn't know it, behind that compulsive and often automatic behavior was the feeling that I was not potent enough. Before I learned about shame, I was not even aware that what I was doing in sex was often driven, disconnected and robotic. I just thought that this was how it was done.

With Amana it changed. She has never been interested in "good sex," she is interested in connection with me. Connecting means not performing or trying to prove anything but being real and open with whatever is there. This gave me a chance to go to the depth of my "castration fears," feeling the emptiness in my genital area, feeling the shame of it and exposing it. In this way, it heals. I can't say that my sexual shame has gone, but I can say that it really isn't an issue anymore. That's the miracle of love.

Having gone through this experience myself helps me to assist other men who are either in shame or trying to run away from it by compensating. Men hate to be rejected sexually because it brings up so much shame. But often, rather than feel and share the shame, they get angry, blame, demand or sink into resignation. These reactions may be habitual and automatic and they shield them from feeling the shame that the rejection has provoked. From a space of being shame-based, it feels almost intolerable to feel the pain of being sexually rejected. A couple we worked with were having sexual problems mostly because the man often felt rejected sexually. But rather than share the insecurities that came up for being rejected, he would blame her for not being open, not being sexy, for being repressed, and for not making herself attractive.

Women may also have shame simply because they feel sexual and enjoy sex. I (Amana) remember years ago being in a relationship where the man would reject me whenever I came to him initiating sex. He would only be open if he initiated the intimacy. Otherwise he would pull away. This opened up deep shame about my sexuality and about being "too much." Many women are conditioned to wait and be passive. When the passion begins to awaken and then is rejected by the man it can be devastating. It takes a lot of courage to move through this rejection, feel the shame and come to the place of knowing inside that there is nothing wrong with passion and with enjoying sex.

Some men may be threatened by this passion but that doesn't make it wrong. We don't have to hold back our energy just because it provokes shame and insecurity in a man. Of course, if we become more expressive and initiating with our sexuality, we also have to be willing to risk being rejected. When that happens, it can trigger deep feelings of feeling "dirty," "sluttish," or unattractive and undesirable. This is particularly strong if we have been conditioned that sex is bad or that a woman should be reserved and hold back her passion. It helps to realize that all this comes from life-negative, repressive ideas held by society and perhaps by our parents as well.

Shame About Your Body

You can also have deep shame about your body and your genitals. At a workshop, Peter, one of the participants, was sitting at dinner with a group of other participants. One of the women was talking about a man she was intimate with whose penis was so small that she couldn't feel him when he was inside, which made her feel unsatisfied sexually. Peter didn't say anything at the time, but this comment triggered him because he had always felt shame about the size of his penis. That evening when we came together in the hall, he had the courage to talk about this episode to the whole group. But even when all the other women said that for them the size of a man's penis had nothing to do with their sexual satisfaction, it was still hard for him to accept that there was not something basically wrong with him because his penis was not as large as he wanted it to be.

In the same workshop, a woman admitted that she felt terribly ashamed of her body — she felt that her breasts were too small, that her hips were not big enough and her legs were too fat. She was even ashamed to be naked in front of her boyfriend of many years. She felt that she had to make sure he was always totally satisfied in their lovemaking — otherwise she was afraid he would leave her. When we asked her why she imagined her boyfriend loved her, she could not think of a single good reason. We suggested that she give him a call and ask him directly why he was with her. When her boyfriend received the call, at first he was taken aback and was only able to say a few things that came to his mind. But for the next three days, he kept sending her text messages with more reasons why he loved being with her.

Shame is hard of hearing. But even so, she came each morning with a bigger smile on her face. When you are in shame and you are taken over by unworthiness, it is hard to imagine why anyone would love you. But love is a powerful force and when it comes in a sincere and honest way, it can even penetrate the thickest wall of shame.

Because of Shame, You Invite Abuse Or Become An Abuser

Sometimes your shame is so great that you tolerate or even invite abuse. Anna, a woman in her thirties, was with a man who regularly beat her, was violent sexually, and frequently made love to other women. She knew that it was not healthy for her to stay with him but she could not leave him. Whenever she tried, she would come back. Her father had also abused both her and her mother physically. She was deeply conditioned to believe that this is how men treat women. She had such low self-esteem and so much shame that she could not imagine being treated in another way.

Rather than see that her partner was disturbed, she idealized him and she blamed herself for being abused. She would tell us repeatedly about all the good sides of her man — his qualities of strength and his good looks. We could see that she was not ready to see him as he actually was. From the space of shame, you easily make choices that are not supportive to your being. Yet over time, she began to understand that this belief about how she and women in general deserve to be treated was a symptom of her shame and came from how she and her mother were treated in the past.

Shame is also the root of abusive behavior. Mark had been physically abused by his father and carried much rage inside. He found that in his relationships with women, he behaved much as his father did toward his mother — abusive, violent, sexually aggressive, demanding and irritable much of the time. He came to us to work with himself because he was beginning to feel the pain of what he was doing and was feeling remorse that his violence was out of control.

Over time, exploring the shame and the fear inside, he discovered that his rage was a cover for deep feelings of helplessness. If he allowed himself to relax, he felt that anyone could abuse him just the way his father did. He also discovered that he felt profoundly insecure about his sexuality, and that if he could not prove to the woman how potent he was, he thought he would never be loved. Becoming aware of this underlying insecurity and being willing to feel the helplessness has made him feel better about himself, and the rage is slowly disappearing.

Facing The Shame

The deeper you go in intimacy, the harder it becomes to hide your shame from yourself or your partner. This is one of the reasons many people avoid intimacy. When you have many partners and change frequently from one person to another, it may be possible to hide behind a mask of performance, to hide behind the excitement of new sex and the thrill of seduction and conquest. You can also hide from your shame if you keep yourself in isolation (which is the main reason we isolate). It takes courage to admit you have sexual shame. But it is also a doorway to deeper intimacy and love when you drop your masks and sink into accepting the depth of your insecurities.

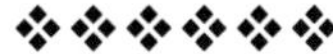

Chapter 6
"You Have to Be There for Me!" How the Regressed Child Shows Itself in Sex

There is a part of you that is primarily concerned with getting what it wants and does not take into consideration the feelings and sensibilities of the other person. This part of you is called, "The Regressed Child." It's actually a regressed adult behaving like a child. When you're taken over by this part, you can be reactive, demanding, entitled, defensive, moody, withheld, emotional, angry, violent, begging, vengeful, controlling, manipulative, righteous, judgmental, critical or depressed, collapsed and resigned. It can even show itself in caretaking, where the child, disguised as an adult, is behaving responsibly and caring but underneath wanting to be taken care of. You often don't realize when you are taken over by the regressed child, because it is so compelling, automatic and unconscious. As with everything else that we have talked about so far, your sex life provokes this part of you strongly and it is good to understand more about it.

A client of ours is a charming, attractive man in his early forties. He complained to us that women leave him after they have been dating for only a short time, and he wants to know the reason. We suggested that he ask this question to the woman he was with most recently. When he asked her, she told him that he was nice and sweet and attractive but as soon as their relating became sexual, she pulled away because she felt that he started behaving like a hungry puppy. This energy made her not want to make love to him because she felt that she was having sex with a needy little boy rather than with a man.

Another client of ours was recently rejected by the woman he had been with for five years. He was not aware why she left him, but he told us that it didn't matter anyway because "the relationship had run its course and it was time for both of us to move on."

Later, when we met her and asked her why the relationship had ended, she said, "He always needed to be in control. When we met, I was impressed with his wisdom and how evolved he was spiritually. But later, I began to see that this was a power game of his. He played the guru/teacher/therapist all the time with me. He wanted to show me how to make love 'spiritually.' And after awhile, I just couldn't stand it anymore." His role as the superior, evolved one is just another face of the regressed child.

Sex is an arena for the regressed child acts out because it is an area where you *want.* You may not know *what* you want or even *that* you want, but you *want.* The problem is not that you have a regressed child (we all do); the problem is that you are not aware of when and how it acts.

> *When our sexuality becomes contaminated with our regressed child, it can sabotage not only the sexuality but the relationship as well. It kills the sexual energy, causes resentment in our partner and feeds our own unwillingness to grow up.*

When you begin to become conscious of how this part of you shows itself in your lovemaking, everything changes. Let's look at some of the common ways this regressed child shows itself and how it affects your sexuality.

The Hungry Penis and the Hungry Vagina — Our Insensitivity in Sex

It's understandable that when you are focused on getting your needs met, you often fail to be sensitive to or in tune with your partner. One couple, Andrea and Peter, came to us because they were having difficulties, particularly in their sexuality.

Andrea explained, "I'm pushing him away because I feel that he's too demanding, too fast, too full of expectations, and it turns me off.

Peter answered, "I admit it's true. I am full of expectations, but it's because she is always rejecting me sexually. And the more she rejects me, the hungrier I get. You know, it wasn't like this when we first got together. She was a sexual animal. In fact, often I felt that I could never satisfy her. I even felt that sometimes when we made love, she was almost raping me."

Andrea countered, "I might have been voracious in the beginning, but now it's him that can never seem to get enough. I feel used, like I am supposed to fill a hole inside for him. And I don't want to make love that way."

Peter said, "That's what I felt with you too. Like I was servicing you.

They had much resentment for each other because of this behavior, but as the session progressed they were able to see that they were both using sex to express and to fill their panic and hunger inside. They were surprised and relieved to understand that this was what was underneath what was happening in their sexuality.

This couple is a good example of what we call, "the hungry penis" or "the hungry vagina." When you come to the other person with a hungry penis or vagina, you are using sex and your partner. You are not in a giving mode; you are in a taking mode. You're using sex in order not to feel deeper places of emptiness, loneliness, insecurity, meaninglessness, pain or fear. You're using sex to escape. Most of us have much neediness and panic inside, and it is common and also human to find ourselves going towards sex to relieve it. The problem is that it's often unconscious and then your partner can easily feel used. Furthermore, from that compulsion to relieve your anxiety and fill the emptiness inside, you can become insensitive, invasive and even abusive toward your partner.

Mary is an attractive woman in her forties. When asked what she expected from men when she made love, she said that she wanted them to be "extremely potent, present, totally there for me, gentle yet firm, soft and hard at the same time and willing to make love to me whenever I want to." Even though she said this with some humor, she admitted that she would get disappointed and ultimately reject the man if he didn't fulfill these needs. After looking deeper into what lies underneath these expectations, she admitted that she actually felt like a very frightened little girl who just wanted to have a man in her life so that she could relax and not have to be so "strong" all the time. Her sexual expectations were a cover for her deep fear of letting a man be the way he is, with all his weaknesses.

You Can Use Sex to Cover Your Wound of Abandonment

As we said, it is understandable that you divert your anxiety, fears and shame into sex. Sex can give relief, closeness, touch or the sense of adventure and conquest, all of which can distract you from feeling the deeper places of fear inside. Sex may relieve your anxiety. But the hungry penis or vagina is covering up deep fears of abandonment that you have not explored and may not even know are there. Also, because of your wound of abandonment and the fear that accompanies it, you can become very demanding in sex.

Steven felt that when he made love to his girlfriend Lisa, she wanted him to be "more of a man." He said that she wanted "...to feel his passionate energy and for him to be so present and strong that she could totally let go."

"Unless I am like that, she tells me that she can't be receptive and feel her femininity. I feel that as a terrible pressure, and I can't live up to her expectations even if I wanted to."

Lisa said, "I want him to make a commitment to be present and in his male energy when he makes love to me. I want a man. It's his potential and his destiny to be a man and to make love with his total presence. Then I can allow myself to rise up to my full potential as a woman - surrendered, open and receptive."

Some of their ideas came from a teacher of sexuality that both of them had studied with, who taught that in true sex, the man's role was to be so present and centered that the woman could totally surrender. We explained that from our understanding, there is a danger of having ideas about how one should be. It can create more pressure, and may prevent people from feeling what is going on at deeper levels. For this couple to be able to love deeply and intimately, he needed to take into consideration his shame and insecurities. She in turn had to consider that her expectations and demands might be a cover for her wound of abandonment.

> *Our wound of abandonment can be triggered whenever we receive a rejection or a loss. It can be triggered every time we feel deprived of love or attention. It can be triggered whenever we feel that our partner is not making love to us they way we would like. Sex is an area where we can be hypersensitive to feeling deprived. Perhaps without knowing it, we link our emotional nourishment and our ego support to sex or closeness. When we get what we want, we feel good— and when we don't, we can become highly disturbed. When the other person withholds sexual energy or rejects our attempts at coming close physically, our wound of abandonment is easily opened.*

I (Krish) had an experience some years ago that strongly brought up this issue for me. Amana, after a meditation retreat, became more introverted and less interesting in sex and connecting. She took more time to be alone and meditate. I was used to her being available, and it was a shock for me to feel that she was gone in the way in which I'd become accustomed. I noticed myself becoming more irritable and critical and also more demanding for intimacy. It took me some months before I could understand what was happening and contain the anxiety and discomfort of the deprivation. As I became more able to contain the frustration, something settled inside. Paradoxically, as I came back to myself, Amana opened up again. (Funny how that happens, isn't it?)

Escaping into Drama

Another way that your regressed child expresses itself in your sexuality is through creating drama. Drama is appealing because it generates intensity and can help the sexuality become more passionate and exciting. A client of ours has for many years habitually been attracted to men who are strong, vibrant and very sexual. She loves the thrill of their power and says that only with these kinds of men can she allow herself to feel vulnerable. But with men who are more sensitive, she takes control and becomes dominant and domineering.

She discovers, though, that with the men she is attracted to, eventually the sexuality becomes excessive, sometimes violent and perverted. When she feels that her man has gone too far in their lovemaking, she feels betrayed. As long as she is in this kind of drama — attracted, sometimes afraid, sometimes turned on, sometimes turned off, sometimes ecstatic and other times in despair — she remains in a regressed state, addicted to the high intensity drama. She doesn't have to grow up and go through what it would be like to have a deepening relationship with a man who is not there just for the thrill of sex.

Escaping into Dependency

When you are being ruled by your regressed child, your relating and your sexuality becomes co-dependent. A couple, Alan and Cynthia, who came to have a session with us, were furious with each other from the moment they entered the room. It took awhile for them even to speak because they were so resentful of each other.

Finally, Alan admitted, "I am furious with Cynthia because she only wants to make love to me when I am in a good space. When I am sad, she rejects me. But I can't be happy all the time! Doesn't love mean that you accept the person no matter what mood he is in?"

Cynthia said, "Aach! I am so so so sick of his complaining, 'hang-dog' energy. Who wants to make love to such a victim! It makes me sick! When we got together, he wasn't like this. He had some juice and I liked to have sex with him. I want to have sex with someone who has energy, not with a wet rag!"

Alan: "Why can't you accept me the way I am?"

Cynthia: "Because, I want a man. I feel betrayed by you. When you're in your victim trip, I don't have a man anymore!"

Once they started into their resentments of each other, it was hard to stop them. Neither of them realized that there was no adult in this relationship — just two entitled, regressed children believing that the other person should fulfill their expectations. This is the royal road toward true suffering. We helped them to see that in this kind of relating, it is not possible to have any harmony, depth or understanding. We worked with helping them to understand that they were in a power struggle (a topic we will take up shortly). The source of the struggle was their expectations, and it was important to go to root of these expectations.

> *The root of expectation is always deeply seated fear of not getting what we need, or not feeling understood, taken in, seen and felt. The difficulty is that is that we get trapped in the idea that the other person should fulfill them.*

Instead, it is important to understand that it is a deep sense of deprivation inside that has been there a long time. There are three understandings that help:

1. This wound has been there a long time;

2. Your partner is going to provoke it because that's what happens in deeper relationships;
3. If you feel and communicate from the place of vulnerability rather than from blame or expectation, you are more likely to get the love you want.

Once we become aware that we are in the control of our regressed child, we have the power to choose to grow up. By seeing how and when our regressed child thinks, acts and feels, we can choose to allow our adult self to run our life instead.

Alan's wound that was being provoked was not feeling understood in his sensitivity and in his pain. Cynthia's was not feeling met in her energy and always feeling inside that she was too much. Of course, both of these had their origin in their childhood. Once having discovered how they were provoking each other and being able to connect to the source, they could share with each other without so much reaction.

Sometimes this drama shows itself by one playing the role of a child and the other playing the role of the parent. (The parent role is still the regressed child but has a fancier cloak.) This dynamic is just as deadly for sexuality. A couple came to a workshop because, after twenty-five years of marriage, they were considering separation. Their sexuality was no longer fulfilling — he was having an affair and they were fighting continually. Before they were a couple, he was a client of hers in psychotherapy. When they fell in love, she allowed what she felt was a reasonable period of time to lapse before they began a relationship and got married. But the power balance between them never changed. She remained the parent and he the child. He looked up to her as his teacher and she lorded this superiority over him.

The one who plays the parent role often finds it comfortable to be the caretaker because it gives him or her a sense of being needed, of power, control and familiarity. The child finds it comfortable because he or she does not have to be responsible, and feels taken care of and safe and/or guided. It is understandable that, given this imbalance, their sex life declined and eventually vanished altogether (it feels incestuous). During the workshop, both of them realized how they had been using this situation to shelter themselves from their wound of abandonment. They were unsure if they could stay together, but both knew that they were ready to create a more mature way of relating and were ready to stop hiding by playing these familiar roles.

It takes a lot of courage to drop the roles and allow the vulnerability of being without our familiar identities. For the one playing the parent role, the challenge is in letting go of control and open to the vulnerability that comes when we allow the other person to do things his or her way. For the one playing the child role, the challenge is to become more responsible and to make decisions, rather than habitually asking for help.

Gaining Some Mastery Over Your Regressed Child

The regressed-child role can kill sexuality and, unless you gain some understanding and mastery of it, eventually it can kill a relationship. The first step is learning to recognize *when* and *how* it shows itself. When you start paying attention to yourself, it becomes easier to notice when your behavior stems from your regressed child. It feels a certain way, and you can learn to watch it in action. You come to know its favorite strategies and see how others respond to you when you are acting from this space. By itself, that observation is transformative because you can see that behaving from the regressed child creates suffering in your life. And it is not a very effective way to get what you want. Part of watching your regressed child in action also includes seeing how it affects the one you love.

Often we are faced with a choice between driving toward getting our own needs met or being sensitive and respectful of our partner.

It is also important to know *why* you act from our regressed child. You react, become emotional, blame, control, criticize, advise, demand, cling, manipulate, beg, rage, cut off, isolate, get depressed or take revenge because you are afraid. You are afraid that you will not get what you need unless you act this way. These behaviors have been there a long time and, at some earlier time, were the basis of your survival. But these behaviors or reactions are no longer based on the here and now. They are based on what you project onto the here and now. Reality today is seldom the same as it was when you developed these behaviors. Slowly, you may begin to see that your reactions are based on the past and may realize that you no longer need to behave in this way.

> *The most important and perhaps the most difficult aspect of gaining mastery over our regressed child is learning to contain the fear and panic that comes up when we are not getting what we want or expect. The behavior of our regressed child is so compelling, unconscious and habitual because it is a primitive effort to reduce anxiety and pain. When we are taken over by our compulsion to relieve our anxiety, there is no space between the trigger (not getting what we want) and our reaction.*

A woman was sharing that when her boyfriend even looked at another woman, she would rage at him. She knew that this behavior was pushing him away but she felt helpless to change this behavior.

We asked her, "What happens in your body when you notice your boyfriend's attention wavering to another woman?"

She responded, "I feel agitated, disturbed, anxious, and can hear thoughts entering my mind that he will leave me because I don't deserve to be loved. I just can't stay with these feelings, they are too much."

As long as we guided her and supported her, she could find the space inside to feel her anxiety and contain it. But she doubted that she could do it on her own.

It takes practice to be able to contain anxiety. You may need some guidance in the beginning. But it is very helpful to know that through learning to contain frustration and anxiety you grow in strength, wisdom and depth, and build a foundation for love. When you commit to learning to contain your fears rather than acting them out on your partner, it begins a process of profound transformation.

As part of a structure to help people build the ability to contain anxiety, disappointment, frustration and pain, we ask them to write down situations that could come up in their life that they simply cannot deal with. They mention situations like rejection, criticism, humiliation, stress or failure. Almost always, when we explore more deeply, they discover that they already are facing these situations in their lives. The difficulty is that they are telling themselves that they can't cope with these situations. It is the regressed child talking. This idea deprives them of the ability to realize that they *can* face them.

Thoughts are powerful. As long as you have the idea that there are certain situations that you simply cannot deal with, you are approaching life with a closed fist. When you remove that idea from your minds, you can open your palms and learn to receive and embrace what life brings. It is amazing how much more strength you find inside when your palms are open. It is surprising how much inner space you discover inside when you *accept* that an essential part of growing up and finding your power is facing your fears and being open to what life brings. Each of us has our pet fears, and usually they are precisely what we need to face.

Since I (Krish) achieved the ability to understand more about how my regressed child thinks and acts, I keep a closer watch. I can feel when he takes over because it feels so different in my body, and my thoughts often have an edge of fear to them. Of course, that is not obvious at first. It took some investigation to see that judging, blaming, expecting and reacting are driven by fear — but now I can *feel* it. By becoming more aware of my regressed child, I can say honestly that this part of me no longer to run my life or my relationships. And I think that it is probably the reason that I am able to sustain a deep and loving relationship with Amana.

> *It is vital for building love to understand that it is not our partner's role to make us feel better and to relieve our anxiety and fear. We are basically alone and whatever we receive from another person in the way of love and companionship is a gift.*

This knowing paves the way for a healthy and mature relationship between two adults. You cannot expect your regressed child to understand this higher perspective, but you are not only the regressed child. You may still react from your regressed child, but at any time you can come back to yourself and realize that this part of you has momentarily taken control of your life. The willingness to stay with the frustration, pain and anxiety is how you build inner space, containment, centering and peace. It is also how you build trust with your partner.

Steps for Gaining Mastery Over Our Regressed Child

1. Begin to Recognize When You Are Behaving Like A Regressed Child.
2. Begin to Feel What It Feels Like To Be A Regressed Child.
3. Begin to Identify the Strategies and Behaviors of Your Regressed Child.
4. Ask Yourself, "How These Behaviors Affect Those Around Me?"
5. Ask Yourself, "What Is The Fear That Is Causing Me to Behave Like a Regressed Child Right Now?"
6. Tell Yourself, "I Have The Capacity To Contain This Fear."
7. Ask Yourself, "What Would Help Me To Contain It?"

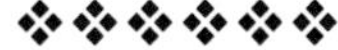

Chapter 7
"Love Games or War Games?" How Power Struggles Poison Our Sex Life

As you get closer to another person, it is almost predictable that emotional issues will develop as the other person provokes your wounds. This is especially strong when you're not happy with who you are or how you are living our life. When you're unwilling to feel the pain or fear that the other person provokes, you move into covering up your feelings with masks or roles.

> *Power struggles are ways that we jockey for control, dominance and position, the ways we need to be right and feel right, the ways we judge others or fight with others because it feels too threatening to be vulnerable. We call this behavior "war games."*

The longer you're with someone, the more you get under each other's skin. Then you act out your frustrations and anxiety on each other. You get jealous. You discover aspects of the other person's personality that you don't like and want to change. You belittle each other. You try to control the other person by becoming his or her teacher, guru, therapist, mother or father. You compete with each other or feel threatened if the other person changes, becomes more alive, more sexual, more angry or more vulnerable. You want the other person to take care of you. You expect the other person to behave and be the person you want him or her to be, perhaps even the person you *imagined* them to be in the beginning.

You judge, criticize, analyze, manipulate and deceive the other person because you want things to be the way you want them to be. You may even have ideas about what the other person should give you, especially in sex, and it may not be what you are getting. You become dishonest and try to cover your dishonesty in different ways. You become resentful and then take revenge in hidden ways. You become aggressive and dominating or passive and withholding. You intimidate your partner in different ways. You play like a child expecting the other person to take care of you, solve your problems, relieve your fears and anxieties, or answer your questions. Or conversely, you play like a parent who is in charge, caretaking and needed.

A woman reported in a session that she was suffering because, "A man with whom I had a hot and passionate seven month affair left me and went back to his wife."

"What was the reason that the affair ended?" we asked.

"He found me too demanding and too needy."

On further exploration, we discovered that she has been married for fifteen years and has two children.

"I had the affair because my husband is a boring lover," she told us.

"What do you mean by boring?" we asked.

"He's not creative, passionate or sensitive when we make love."

"Have you ever worked with your husband to try and improve your sex life by taking sessions together or attending sexuality workshops?"

"I don't think that he will ever change.

"Did you tell your husband about the affair?" we asked.

"No, definitely not! If I did, he would leave me."

In our work, we often encounter people who have grown accustomed to living in relationship with much dishonesty. In any long-term relationship, there is much potential for power struggles to develop, and if two people aren't growing together in love and understanding, the power games *will* develop and will *not* get resolved. In fact, when the power struggles are unconscious and/or unresolved, they build and begin to dominate how you relate and how you make love. Eventually, they become pure poison to the love and the sexuality. It takes respect and sensitivity toward yourself and toward each other to build love. It takes a constant willingness to maintain that respect and sensitivity. Power games erode the delicate trust that two people can build together.

The Roots of Power Games

A woman in a workshop shared that she had recently broken up with her boyfriend because he had become sexually violent. When we explored more deeply with her, she confessed that she had a pattern of tormenting men with her demands and her criticisms and felt more comfortable fighting than allowing them to see her vulnerability. She knew that this fear dated back to her conflictual relationship with her father but she still did not see how to change this pattern. (Often we use the discovery of our childhood wounds only as an excuse to continue to justify our patterns and our power games.) Because of her fears of opening and being vulnerable, she found it safer and more familiar to engage in power games with her men. She related with strategies of revenge, withholding, and being sexually demanding. She would torment them to the point that they would become violent, and then she would feel abused and leave. These experiences then reinforced her belief that it is not safe to open and be vulnerable.

- We play power games because we're afraid that if we become vulnerable, we may be hurt, abused or rejected.
- We get into power games because we're insecure of our personal power and our self-identity is filled with shame and feelings of inadequacy.

- We struggle for power because we feel that if we don't, we will be dominated, controlled or lose face in our own eyes or in the eyes of the other person.
- We also engage in power games when we forsake our own vision and our own creativity for the sake of a relationship.

It takes courage to open your vulnerabilities, your hurts and your fears to each other and it takes risk to stand your ground in moments when you need to. It is easier, more automatic, more familiar and more habitual to fight or pull away.

A client of ours was offered a job that he had wanted for years, but his partner complained that it would mean spending a fair amount of time traveling and being away from her. He hesitated to take the offer and asked for six months to decide. But he noticed that he was becoming increasingly depressed and their sexuality faded. Finally, after some inner struggle and encouragement from us, he decided to take the job. By following his energy, their relating and their sexuality improved dramatically.

Often, you don't want to face your deeper fears and vulnerabilities, share them with your partner, and learn what is behind your conflicts. You prefer to fight, perhaps because you know no other way. Besides, there may be a certain thrill to fighting. Perhaps you enjoy the challenge and the excitement of combat. Often, when two people have unresolved power struggles, they may find themselves in the kind of sexual relationship in which they fight and then make up with more passionate lovemaking — "make-up sex." It's the *drama* that turns them on. But that kind of arrangement is painful, hurtful and exhausting, and it gets old quickly. It is a big shift when you begin to open and expose your vulnerability and traumas to yourself and to your partner. Until you do, your relating and your sex become dominated with war games.

I (Krish) know from my own experience that when I'm hurt, my first instinct has been to blame or cut off. And when this hurt involves sex, these instincts are even stronger. Over the years, I've learned that to react in this way just perpetuates my own pain as well as the pain of the other person. With Amana, it's been safe to open because she too is not interested in staying in a power game. We short-circuit them quickly because we both feel the pain when we are disconnected from each other.

Sometimes it takes a little time to be with yourself before it is time to come together again and share openly. When you come to your partner with a charge, it is difficult or impossible to communicate. We have used a simple technique to reconnect that we describe at the end of the chapter. It is a technique that we adopted from the work of Harville Hendricks. [See references]. Here it is in brief: First, you ask if the other person has the space to listen. Then you make an attempt to share without blame or expectation. The other person simply listens and then reflects back what he or she has heard to make sure it is correct. Then the listener has time to share in the same way. It took some practice but over time, we have learned to do this well and it has worked to prevent resentments from building between us. It is extremely important for love and trust to flow freely that both partners have the willingness to keep cleaning anything that comes in the way.

Some Examples of Common War Games

A couple that we worked with seemed to others to be mild mannered and sweet with each other, but when they were alone with each other they fought incessantly. He hated her behaving like a little girl and she hated his acting like a dominating, raging male chauvinist. She alternated between going into shock with his tyrannical behavior or fighting back. Her retaliation of choice was sleeping with other men. When he finally lost control one day and hit her, she retaliated by refusing to make love to him. And so it went.

Another couple we worked with fought because he insisted that he could not be a man unless she became more vulnerable, receptive and open. She felt that until he behaved like a man, she didn't feel safe enough to be vulnerable and open. Sexually, he felt that he could not be empowered as a man until she became more receptive. And she felt the same in reverse. Finally, she went off with another man, had an affair. Then she told her partner that with this new man, she could feel totally receptive because he was present and centered in their lovemaking and that allowed her to open. She just needed a man to be "totally in his energy" for her to open. His reaction to her revenge was naturally to cut off from her.

> *War games escalate. Waiting for the other to stop, to become vulnerable and open, is just another war game. Power struggles are run by fear. To short-circuit our war games, we have to connect with the fear that is driving them and take the risk to feel and expose the fear.*

The Angry Penis or the Angry Vagina

In a training, a woman shared that she felt her husband was using his penis as a weapon when he made love to her and that he was acting out his anger with her and perhaps women in general in this way. Sex can bring up deeply repressed anger that we may carry toward the opposite sex. Many of us have resentments that go all the way back to childhood with our opposite sex parent — resentments for being invaded, disrespected, or even abused. Often you're not aware that you carry these resentments but they can suddenly surface while making love.

We call this "the angry penis" or "the angry vagina." A man in a recent workshop had been the emotional lifeline for his mother during his childhood. He admitted that sometimes while having sex, he just wanted to hurt the woman with his penis. He wanted to take revenge or prove to her that he was the boss and she should do exactly as he said.

Another participant told us that whenever he saw a woman he found attractive, he would imagine undressing her and having sex with her in hard and violent ways. He also told us that he had been compulsively drawn to watching pornography since age twelve, and that in the past he had had relationships with women that were based entirely on sex. The sex they had was so hard and violent that after some time he could not take it anymore.

All of these are manifestations of the angry penis. His mother was an unhappy and tense person who had a painful and disconnected relationship with his father. She felt that men were violent and sexually obsessed and gave him the message that sex was disgusting and shameful.

When we ask participants to express what their angry penis or their angry vagina is saying, they make statements such as:

Women:

- "Now you're mine!"
- "You won't get me!"
- "You can never give me enough!"
- "Come and get me and then I'll show you!"
- "I won't let you in!"
- "I will eat you!"
- "I'm not going to let you go!"
- "I can do whatever I want with you!"

Men:

- "I'm not going to satisfy you!"
- "I'm going to satisfy you like no man has ever done before!"
- "I want to rape you!"
- "I want to kill you!"
- "I want to dominate you!"
- "I'm going to fuck you forever!"
- "You're mine!"
- "I want you to feel my power!"
- "I want you to feel how much you want me!"

Even though most of us have some of these feelings of rage and resentment inside, sex is not the appropriate place for acting it out. Sex is not an avenue to cathart our anger, rage or resentment because we can easily traumatize each other and damage the trust between us.

It is healthier for the person and for the relationship to work out this energy in a therapeutic environment. That's why it's important to understand where it comes from. Much of the time, the angry penis is a compensation for feeling repressed, castrated and humiliated as a child. Men have a deep wound of feeling castrated. It is linked, consciously or unconsciously, to their mother — and, collectively, to all women. They may experience the castration wound as an emptiness in the genital area. But rather than feel the emptiness or the fear, they may move into compensating. They perform to prove their power or move into violence because it may feel as if the woman is responsible for this feeling of impotence.

Andrew shared that when he made love, he could feel the anger and the desire to "fuck the woman's brains out," as he put it. When we asked him to go deeper into this energy and say what came up, he said, "I want to prove to the woman that I am potent. I want to dominate the woman. I want to feel my power over the woman and feel that she is my sex slave. I want to feel that she is both attracted and also afraid of me." Andrew's father was in the military and regularly abused him physically as a child. He was still feeling the humiliation his father caused him as well as carrying his father's rage in his body.

A man shared with us about his time with his now ex-wife, who was an alcoholic. They would make love when she was drunk, and they would play with bondage and other sex games. Now, when he looks back, he realizes that he betrayed himself by participating in this kind of sex. It was a way of acting out, in a dysfunctional way, the unexpressed rage that they had for each other. Since that time, he has started an intensive program of workshops and individual therapy and is working with his rage. Now that he has found another way to express his anger, he can't imagine ever making love in that way again.

> *It takes courage for men to allow the feelings of impotence and emptiness in the genitals and even more courage to expose that to a woman. It helps to see the futility of the ceaseless efforts to prove potency and to see that these compensations usually only bring less self-respect and dignity. When we drop behind the power games, allowing ourselves to feel the castration wound, it is a doorway to real strength, a strength that comes from openness and relaxation rather than performance, pushing or violence.*

Many women carry deep resentments toward their father or other male adults from their past who may have been insensitive and even invasive toward them. A woman came to a workshop and began complaining from the start. The food was terrible, the place was ugly and uncomfortable and there were too many people in the room for her to open up. When we asked her some questions about herself, she became enraged at how superficial the questions were and how out-of-touch with her we were.

But with time, we reached the source of her rage. She discovered some years back that her father had abused her sexually and he refused to admit it. She maintained a relationship with him because, "He is my father," but pushed away any man who tried to come close to her. As she was quite physically stunning, she had many offers, but she found some excuse to reject, sooner or later, all the men who showed interest in her — or even those she spent time with.

As she talked, she became more and more vulnerable and honest.

"In the past," she said, "I had no trouble letting men in and no trouble with sex. Now, when a man comes near me, all I feel is rage."

We explained that her rage was to be expected, and aggravated by maintaining a relationship with the father who remained in denial and would not feel the pain and damage he had caused her.

Even women who have not suffered from sexual abuse have good reasons to feel rage toward men — not the least of which is centuries of domination. This rage is in the female collective. This energy is powerful and can easily surface while making love. As with men, it can come up as a desire to dominate, perhaps even to cause pain to the partner. Or, it may show itself as a total lack of sexual feeling. However, whether with men or with women, it is important to recognize the hostility and resentment that we harbor inside and to find more creative ways to work with it than acting it out in the bedroom (or any other room where we might make love, for that matter).

Dropping Power Games

Bearing in mind that dropping power games is a process that takes time, we would like to outline what we consider to be the steps that we need to take.

a) Recognizing the War Game

A first step for dropping war games is noticing and feeling when you are in one. One sign that you are in a war game is to notice that your focus is on trying to influence the other person, or his or her behavior in some way. There is also a certain sensation connected to a power game that you can feel in the body. If you pay attention, you can feel the violence in your energy and the obsessive way that your behavior and thoughts are directed toward the other person. Also, when you are in a war game, there is an obsessive and irrational feeling that it is not safe to be vulnerable. It also helps to become aware of your own particular power games and observe how habitual and automatic they are.

While noticing and watching your war games is a big step towards transformation, you also have to reach a point in your life when you recognize that they are old destructive patterns that only serve to push other people away. Power struggles hurt, and when you play them you pay a big price. You feel separate, hostile, unloving, unloved and isolated. At first, you may want to justify your anger and your defense when you have felt wronged. But at a certain point, you may be able to see that the price of staying protected is too big a price to pay. You may need time to lick your wounds and cool down. But then, if the willingness is there to go beyond the power struggles, you can drop our pride and come to your partner to make a sincere effort to resolve the conflict.

b) Feeling and Exposing the Fear and Shame Behind the War Game

A second step toward resolving war games is to feel and share the fear and shame that is behind them. If you are willing to open to your vulnerability — to your trauma, fears and insecurities — you can undermine your habitual power games by dropping below them. This not only involves recognizing that you have fears and shame — and understanding where they come from — but it also includes a sincere willingness to feel and expose them to your partner. The fear underneath the power game may be the fear that your partner will leave you or take advantage of your vulnerability. The shame may be that you don't feel worthy, lovable, or proud of yourself as a man or as a woman.

> *When we are not proud of ourselves, it is difficult to allow someone close to us. Power games are the way we keep the other person away.*

c) Learning to Set Boundaries

You fight when you're not confident in your ability to set limits and affirm your boundaries. You're afraid to set limits because of the terror of provoking the other person's anger, hurt or displeasure, and because of your fear to be alone. Sandra has been in a relationship with a man for seven months, but tells us that she is making love with him in ways that are not satisfying for her. He mostly wants oral sex and she feels that this is no longer what she wants. But she's too afraid of losing him to object. Rachel has been with her husband for ten years, but she's also no longer satisfied with how they make love. She wants to take more time to allow melting to happen, and not to be so focused that he would not accept it or understand what she wants.

> *When we reach a point where aloneness feels better than compromising our integrity, and we realize that we can withstand our partner's anger, rejection or displeasure, then we can slowly learn to set boundaries.*

At this point, something changes dramatically in your life. The rage and the desire for revenge begin to pass. Initially, there is too much fear and shock to have the presence of mind to say no to what does not feel right. Most of us have been conditioned to say yes and to maintain harmony because of the fear of punishment or losing love. And then you betray yourself and your body. When you betray yourself, it makes you feel deep shame and out of this shame you betray ourselves even more. It is a vicious circle.

As you start to heal from the shame, often rage arises toward those you have betrayed yourself with and also rage towards yourself for betraying yourself. This is a phase you have to pass through. As your shock heals and you are able to stay in touch with yourself and with your body experience, it becomes easier and easier to say "no" moment-to-moment when something doesn't feel right. And then you can choose to stop betraying yourself and your body and face whatever consequences that action may have. This brings an immense sense of dignity and self-respect.

d) Learning to Feel and Listen to the Other Person's Hurt

A couple who came to see us were fighting and were going back and forth between deciding if they wanted to be together or not. They both felt deeply misunderstood and acted out their hurt with anger toward each other. When we asked them to share their hurt, at first they both launched into blaming the other person.

She said, "You never create enough time for us to be together!"

He responded, "You don't understand all the responsibilities I am facing with work, taking care of my child, and also making time for you." (The child he referred to was from a previous marriage.)

But when we asked them if they were willing to *listen*, to feel the hurt behind the other person's anger, they both relaxed. Both said that what they most wanted was to feel listened to and taken in. Gradually their hearts softened and they learned to listen to each other.

Often what drives your war games is the desperation that you want to be heard. Once you can give that to each other, something profoundly relaxes. Hearing your partner's hurts and needs doesn't mean that you're obliged to meet those needs. Often, (though naturally not always), once you feel listened to, you feel less compulsion to have all your needs met. You begin to see that wanting the other to fulfill your needs comes from your regressed child. Also, sometimes, you're so triggered and emotional that you don't have the space to listen. Again, your regressed child has taken over and it can take you some time to cool down and get some perspective. But later, you can come together and listen, knowing that your power struggles and conflicts come from fear and insecurity.

Playing Love Games Instead of War Games

War games plant seeds of resentment, anger and loss of trust. Ultimately it is your choice whether you want to make love or make war. It is important to know which is which. Violence, demanding, domination, control, blame, guilting, throwing tantrums, being irresponsible and inconsiderate, telling the other person what to do and how to be... these are all war games. You begin to play love games when you cherish yourself and the one you are with. You love when you are willing to listen to and validate your own hurts without automatically blaming someone else. You love when you are willing to listen to and feel the other person without making yourself wrong. You love when you give respect and freedom both to yourself and to the other person.

A Technique for Dropping Power Games

Step 1: Recognize when you're in a power game or when you feel disconnected, angry or hurt with your partner. You can do this by noticing how being in a power game feels inside — how it feels in your body, how you speak and how you act.

Step 2: Take time to be with yourself and feel what this brings up for you. Allow yourself to feel the hurt, the fear or the insecurity that is behind the anger or the game.

Step 3: When you feel that you are able to approach your partner without blame, expectation or the desire to change him or her, ask if he or she has the space to listen to you. Keep your sharing to ten minutes.

Step 4: Share your hurt; fear or insecurity while the partner simply listens. For instance, "When this happened (or when you did or said this), I felt." "And it reminds me of an earlier time when..." If you notice that you are blaming or wanting the other person to change, recognize that you are back in a power game. Start again. Your partner can reflect back what you have said and you can say if he or she heard you correctly.

Step 5: Now invite your partner to speak, "I would like to hear how it is for you." (Without blame, expectation or wanting to change you) and it is your turn to listen. Again, limit the sharing to ten minutes.

❖❖❖❖❖❖

Chapter 8
"I Can't Let You In and I Can't Keep You Out." The Challenges of Opening

Sometimes while making love you open profound inner spaces in your being and can even have experiences of ecstasy. These experiences are possible without being in touch with or exposing your vulnerability to yourself or to your partner. This may be one of the attractions of having multiple partners because there is less of a risk of exposure and vulnerability.

But with an intimate partner, it is more complicated. Sometimes lovemaking can lift you to ecstatic spaces and allow you to feel deeply connected to your partner. Other times, as we have described in previous chapters, it takes you deep into your shame and fears. You may feel insecure, awkward, unloved, unlovable, not met energetically, uncared for, abandoned or invaded and come away feeling unnourished, sad or angry.

Many of us underestimate how incredibly sensitive and vulnerable we are. We may be able to relate and have sex in a superficial way that can be exciting and fun but perhaps not deeply nourishing. We have a deep place inside where we seldom let anyone approach us. We call it your "inner sanctum." It is possible, even common, to be with someone for years and never allow them to touch this "inner sanctum."

To make love in a way where our centers truly meet is a risk. Until we have a stronger sense of ourselves, it is difficult to have a deep intimacy and a healthy sexuality.

Because of past traumas, you lost two important qualities. One is the ability to feel your boundaries and set appropriate limits. The second is an inner sense of yourself that is untouched by what others think and what others want or expect from you. When you begin to retrieve these two qualities, it becomes easier to become vulnerable when you make love and even more importantly, you can allow someone into your "inner sanctum."

Relating on the Periphery

When you relate from a space in which you lack an inner sense of self and a sense of your own boundaries, your relating and your sexuality tends to remain superficial and follow specific patterns. To make it simple we are going to look at four distinct relating styles. Each is a different way that you act out your regressed child and prevent your partner and yourself from connecting with your depth of vulnerability.

- *The mystified style* — You lose yourself in the other person.
- *The isolated style* — You keep a distance, never allowing the other person to come too close.
- *The hysterical style* — Your relating and sexuality is full of drama and intensity but little depth and real intimacy.
- *The power style* — Your relating and sexuality is dominated by power games covering up the vulnerability.

1. The Mystified Style

In this style, you act out your regressed child by attempting to find someone to look up to and hopefully take away some of your anxiety. You give away your power and responsibility and you listen to the other person's beliefs and opinions above your own. You allow others to come in indiscriminately because you idealize them. You may easily become disillusioned when the other person falls from grace, and then feel betrayed and resentful that you listened to him or her and followed his or her advice. On a deeper level, you may even be angry with yourself for not having more intelligent boundaries.

Patricia fell in love with a man who was twenty years older and who was in a long-term relationship with another woman. He was wealthy and charismatic, and she felt flattered that he was attracted to her and loved the attention he gave her. He told her from the beginning that it was just a fling for him while his partner was away for two months and that he had no intention of leaving her. Patricia told him that it didn't matter, she wanted to be with him anyway and would enjoy their connection while it lasted. They had a hot and passionate time but, as he had warned her, after two months he ended the affair.

When he left she was devastated, and she disparaged him among all their mutual friends. She felt used and betrayed and could not understand how he could be so insensitive and heartless. She felt that she had allowed him to come closer than any previous man in her life and could not comprehend how someone who had been so intimate with her could possibly just get up and leave. While stronger and more confident in her professional life, when it came to intimacy Patricia easily lost a sense of herself and was not able to see the other person or the situation for what it was.

2. The Isolated Style

In this style, you act out your regressed child by habitually pulling into your cave and keeping a constant distance from those you come close to. Your relating has a quality of coolness and detachment. Christian and Loretta have been married for eight years and have two children. Loretta first came to work with us because of a history of sexual trauma, but she was also unhappy in her marriage. She shared that Christian was deeply introverted and rarely if ever opened himself. He went about his life as if he were in a private cocoon. Even in their lovemaking he was distant and seemingly not present. She had tried to reach him in different ways, and added that, unfortunately, sometimes she became highly emotional and reactive to his distance.

The following year, Christian came to attend a workshop with us. We met a deeply sensitive man who was so shocked and in his own world that he rarely spoke. After the workshop, we did not hear from him for two years. But in the meantime, Loretta told us that he had started to let her in a little more and communicate — although he would quickly retreat again into his own world.

Although this example is somewhat extreme, it shows the essential aspects of this relating style. When you are so isolated from others, especially those most intimate with you, you find a way to seek nourishment that does not involve other people. You may even have contact with your inner sensitivity and with your fears and shame, but you do not allow others to intrude. You may be intensely lonely, but often you are so disconnected from feeling that you are not even in touch with your loneliness. Your tendency, when you relate or make love, is not to be present because being open is terrifying. You do not feel safe to allow someone to touch you inside. You may even choose to avoid relating and sex altogether, or live with another without contact or opening.

And sometimes in this style you avoid relating or contact with others altogether. Such was the case of a young man who came to work with us. He was profoundly shy and frozen. He only spoke when spoken to, and although he was attracted to women he had never made love or even dated. In the guided meditation structures he invariably went very deep, but in the exercises to share himself he had much difficulty. He simply couldn't find the words to express what he was experiencing in his inner world. When we helped him, he was able to say that he stopped relating because since early childhood he felt that no one understood him or even bother to listen.

He judged himself horribly because he was so uncommunicative and felt like a failure. He was trying to figure out what to do with his life but was confused and afraid of disappointing his successful, wealthy and powerful father. He felt lost, lonely and isolated in his life. "What was the point of sharing," he said, "when I am so confused." But as he opened, he could feel that it was easier to talk in an environment where others listened and seemed interested. He gradually found it easier to speak and began to feel a joyfulness inside that he could not remember feeling for a long time. And this is true for all of the relating styles we are describing. When we find the courage to share from our vulnerability, we begin to get the nourishment that we so long for.

3. The Hysterical Style

Edward and Marta have been in a love relationship for three years, and during that time their relating has been punctuated by high drama. She is very demanding of his time and energy and gets upset whenever she feels that she is not getting what she wants. At first, she tells him what she wants, but when she feels that he is not responding the way she wants him to, she gets angry and more insistent. His response to her behavior varies. Sometimes he complies; other times he pushes her away. But in either case, he feels resentful and manipulated. He is too afraid to set clear and loving limits, and when he reacts to her demands with anger it only makes her anxiety worse. Then, they escalate into shouting contests to the point of physical violence. Because both of them have so much fear and neither is at home with him or herself, they easily trigger each other and at the same time, feel deeply misunderstood and betrayed.

In this style, you act out your regressed child by incessantly creating dramas because you are hypersensitive to rejection or disapproval. You engage passionately, but are always on the lookout for and even expect betrayal. You want closeness and contact, but you are highly suspicious that someone will be insensitive to you or unable to fulfill your needs. Your relating and sexuality can swing between feeling love and feeling betrayed. You may open, but always with the condition that the other person will treat you as you expect (which is not really opening at all) — and when he or she doesn't, you close in rage or resignation.

When you feel betrayed, as you invariably will, your mistrust is validated and you become even more convinced that true intimacy and love is impossible. Yet you are convinced that it is the other person's fault that love has failed. He or she is just not sensitive enough to merit your opening and your trust. This style is a perfect setup for sexual war games, alternating between intense passion and intense conflict, between hot "togetherness" and angry distance. Even when people with this behavior share their fears, it is often in a demanding and manipulative way — with the hidden expectation that the other person is going to rescue them.

4. The Power Style

In this style, you're obsessed with finding ways to be in control and have power over the other person. Samuel spent years as a successful lawyer and became wealthy. He had been married and had two children with his wife, but he realized that he had never been in love with her, and eventually they divorced. After that, he spent several years with a girlfriend, but she continually complained of his ongoing affairs and his not allowing her to get close to him. As soon as he felt vulnerable with his girlfriend, he sabotaged the closeness by spending a night with another woman. It's his way of making sure that he has the upper hand.

Peter is a successful workshop leader whose habit with women in the past has been to have short and passionate relationships and then move on. Recently, he has become involved with a woman and feels that, for the first time in his life, he does not want to lose her. This is a huge step for him, but she often gets provoked when he plays the role of the guru, doesn't listen to her, and pretends to hold a monopoly on the "truth." It is still difficult for him to see that he is using this power game to stay in control and stay safe.

In this style, your relating is dominated by positioning and power games. Your boundaries are rigid. You may even delude yourself that you are close to the other person because you have never experienced what true love and closeness really is. In this style, you feel safe because you are not letting anyone come close, and you can remain preoccupied with the games and the strategies. In sex, you disconnect from your vulnerability and make love to feel passion and power. This aloofness and power may seem attractive to the other person at first, but later he or she feels disappointed, frustrated, and even enraged that you don't open.

Another way the "power style" may show is that you play the rescuer. The rescuer is preoccupied with the needs of the other person and ready to give advice at any time. In this way, you don't have to feel your own fears and insecurities. As the helper, teacher or guru, you comfort your ego, but sooner or later you will encounter resentment from those you have this kind of power over because nobody likes to feel dependent and infantilized forever. People who relate from a mystified place fall easy prey to someone in the power style. They get "blinded by the "light" and the power person is more than happy to take advantage of it.

> *All these styles have one thing in common — they are simply different ways of protecting ourselves and not opening. Depending on our emotional makeup, we pick one of these patterns or some combination of them to keep up our wall and prevent someone from penetrating inside. It is also easy to see how these games can play out and eventually sabotage our sexuality.*

The Depth of Your Inner Sensitivity

You may often wonder why it is so difficult to trust someone, why it is so difficult to let someone inside or why, in a relationship (even a long-term relationship), you often feel that the other person is still a stranger. When you have not explored your fears and insecurities and if your focus and energy have been largely directed toward other people or worldly pursuits, you may have little contact or awareness of your inner world and with the depth of your sensitivity.

In an exercise that we do in our work, we ask people what it feels like when they open their innermost, private place to another person. Some are quite unfamiliar with this space inside and have a hard time understanding what we are talking about. Others say that they hesitate to let someone so close because they realize that they themselves don't know this private place. Or, they say that they have never shared it with another person because they wouldn't know how. Still others say that they are afraid to show this to another for fear of being left, invaded, not being taken in, understood or seen. Or, they are afraid that the other person will judge them for what they find. Yet at the same time, many have a deep longing to open to another person in such a profound space of intimacy.

The Loss of The Inner Sense of Self

Normally, your sensitivity is not supported, and therefore it is easily forgotten. When you lose touch with yourself, you lose touch with your center, your core and the sense of yourself. Once you lose this connection, you get lost in the outer experience of self. This is what happened to most of us. This outer experience of self becomes based on roles which you have learned, on attitudes of yourself which you have developed from your past, on what you feel is expected of you or on what you have learned earns you love and recognition.

> *Now, instead of being connected to an inner space that is grounded in intuitive being, we base our sense of self on rigid roles, rules, standards or beliefs and on inner and outer expectations. Our focus and self-esteem is dependent on appreciation or approval from the outside and defined by outer accomplishments.*

We sometimes ask people to say what they consider makes them worthy as a person. Invariably, they begin to list qualities which they think makes them a worthwhile person — qualities like sensitive, intelligent, giving, alive, spiritual and so on. We respond by saying, "Nope, it's all wrong.

You are worthy because you *are, because you exist.* Period." It creates a tremendous amount of stress when you base your self-worth on ideas of how you should be, on other people's opinions, on things or on roles, instead of resting inside yourself. But because of your conditioning, you have come a long way from home. The first step toward coming home again is realizing how much of your energy is focused on the outside. That can motivate you to find another point of reference, something which is grounded in your being and in your natural intelligence. When that becomes a place from which you feel yourself, it becomes easier to allow another person in. Until then, it can be terrifying and fragmenting.

It has been a long but also beautiful journey to find a place inside of me (Krish) where I could feel safe enough to allow true intimacy. I began utterly focused on external reflections as a way to feel and accept myself. But through years of meditation and working with myself, I have gradually come to find myself. That experience has come from learning to listen to my body, which is infinitely wiser than my mind. It has also come from learning to trust a certain inner sense of "right" that is hard to explain in words. As time went on, I came to feel that I could more and more follow an inner flow. It's a place where I and my life happen without the usual habit of driving and pushing. But old habits die hard, and I still have to be vigilant and aware when I get lost in the old ways.

The Loss of Your Personal Boundaries

Without an ability to feel and affirm your personal boundaries, it is very hard to open. Unless you feel the power to say "no" to what does not feel right, it feels dangerous to let someone in. This is especially true when it comes to sex. As a child, you have no protection or boundaries. In your state of innocent trust, you allow others to enter indiscriminately. Most often, the people who raised you had also learned to disconnect from themselves. Because of this, they entered into your precious inner space without respect for its exquisite sensitivity and without an understanding for what you needed for support.

> *As a result of this intrusion, two things happened. The first was that we were distracted from our natural being and abandoned our grounding in this space. The second is that we carry the memory of people whom we loved and whom we trusted entering into our private space without respect. We develop the belief, either consciously or unconsciously, that it is no longer safe to allow anyone so close.*

A child does not have the resources or the understanding to set limits. When invasion happens without the ability to set limits and say "no," you go into a state of shock. You freeze and dissociate, desperately trying to find a way to be safe even as the invasion happens. But as a result of these invasions, you often lose a sense that you have a separate space or body that you can defend. Today, partly because you did not learn to set limits, and partly out of the hunger for love and attention or the fear of punishment, anger or disapproval, you continue to allow your boundaries to be invaded. Much of the time, you do not even know that you have been invaded because you are so used to being treated this way. You have shrunk your space inside the body to the point where someone can even abuse your body and you don't feel it as an invasion. Because of this, the thought of saying "no" may not even arise.

While discussing this topic in a workshop, one woman shared that she has always believed that the only way to get a man was to offer him sex the way he wanted. All her adult life, she has overrun her own boundaries and her body. A man said that he has been a compulsive pleaser all of his life. Even the thought of saying "no" brings up so much anxiety that he dismisses the idea as quickly as it arises. When your boundaries become damaged, your sense of self fragments. You lose your grounding, your center, and your sense of safety. Either you have rigid and impenetrable boundaries or you have no boundaries at all. When you can no longer choose consciously and clearly if, when and how you want to allow someone to enter, you do not have real intimacy. If you allow someone to come inside without clear discrimination, you will resent that person when he or she does not treat you as you would like. And if you shut people out totally, you have the pain of isolation.

> *Once the pain of betraying ourselves becomes greater than the fear of what could happen if we set our limits, we regain our dignity. Yes, there is a fear of punishment, disharmony, hurting the other person — and, worst of all, rejection and loneliness. But the pain of disrespecting ourselves is worse. By taking the smallest of steps to say "no" when something does not feel right, especially in lovemaking, we develop new habits and reclaim the dignity we have lost.*

People tell us over and over again that once they began to risk setting limits, the reaction they received was nothing like they imagined.

Rediscovering Yourself

The process of coming home begins when you start to see that something is missing. What is missing is inside of you, not something from the outside. You notice that in many ways you have been living your life as a robot, as a slave to identities, roles and beliefs that you have taken for granted. When you take a closer look, you may begin to question the beliefs you were given and have lived by for so long. You may even begin to see that some or all of the values we have been holding on to are not true for you anymore. This insight can spread to all the roles, beliefs and identities that you hold. As they fall away, you may even have a crisis of identity. This crisis can be frightening and disruptive, but it is also highly positive as it shakes you loose from the false and opens you up to the world of the real.

A participant in one of our training sessions shared with us that what motivated him to join the training was that he had fallen into a deep depression. Married for twenty years and the father of three teenage children, he was living an affluent suburban life until four years ago. Then something changed. Everything that he had known seemed empty and colorless to him. He no longer felt sexual attraction for his wife; he quit his job, and he went to see doctors and psychiatrists to find out what was going on. After being thoroughly checked out medically without result and having tried several different antidepressants, nothing helped. His wife wanted a divorce.

The only activity that gave him some degree of happiness was being with his children. He booked our training in the hope that an alternative approach to healing which we offered might work. He was describing a profound identity crisis. His old life no longer gave him meaning. He was in a painful gap and most often, it is precisely this kind of a crisis which motivates us to find ourselves.

> *An essential step toward self-discovery is to take time away from the outer world of fixed roles, power games, the search for respect and approval, success and security.*

Often life events and experiences force this shift on us without a conscious choice as it did with the man in our workshop. At first when this happens, you usually begin to touch deep fears that you have avoided to feel. And you may encounter profound feelings of meaninglessness and sadness because you have begun to see the falseness of how you have lived and what you have believed in. If you go deeper in your discovery, knowing that this is an integral part of the journey inside, you will start to encounter a new sense of meaning based on feeling a part of something much more profound and nourishing than whatever you have felt previously. Generally, you need to face the pain you have been running away from to reach this inner place of nourishment. But as you go deeper into this process, your creativity begins to flow out of a connection to your inner self, and it has a different quality to it. It is less driven and obsessive and more flowing and natural.

A New Way of Relating

Once you have begun to discover yourself and become more confident in setting limits, relating with yourself and others changes profoundly. You appreciate yourself and others in a totally different way. You begin to sense the exquisite sensitivity and delicacy of each person and for the process of intimacy. When you are opening to another person and as trust and sensitivity deepens, you begin to share the most intimate inner spaces with each another without any words or any kind of doing. It just happens.

However, to allow someone into this delicate space, you need to feel a certain groundedness in your being. This groundedness grows as you begin to live more in tune with your truth. Here are some things that, from our experience, help build grounding in your being:

- To become more honest with yourself and in your relating;
- To honor your own needs enough so that you stop betraying your body and yourself;
- To surround yourself with people and environments where you feel loved and supported;
- To express your creativity and other aspects of your essential life energy in spite of your fears of rejection or failure;
- To begin to live your life in a way that you are proud of. This includes how you relate, what you eat, how you act and how you spend your day.

Once we appreciate how sensitive and how vulnerable we really are, a deeper meeting happens only when we respect how fragile the trust is which we develop with another person and how easy it is to damage the delicate trust. When we do something that damages this delicate trust, we can repair it, but only once we value the depth of the other person's sensitivity and how delicate the bond is between two people at this level of intimacy.

This means feeling the hurt and the pain your actions may have caused the other person. At this level of sensitivity, you begin to understand what love is. Unless you honor this sensitivity and nourish it, you destroy the love.

It is possible for two people to meet in profound trust and respect. But this can only happen once you take the fears and insecurities of the other person (as well as your own) into your heart and safeguard those fears as if they were a great treasure to be protected with the greatest care. It takes time and a deep willingness to feel and understand yourself before you feel safe enough to share deeply with another person. By becoming aware of the depth of your sensitivity and preciousness, you slowly become acquainted with your own vulnerability. You respect yourself enough to decide if, when and how much you would like to open to another.

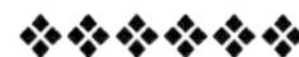

Part III

The Healing

Chapter 9
Becoming Sensitive to Yourselves
How Sex and Vulnerability Can Come Together

When fear and insecurity arise in lovemaking, it's a natural reaction to want to avoid sex, to not be present in sex, or perhaps to find a new partner who does not bring up these feelings. Many couples we have worked with, not understanding how sex changes as intimacy deepens, have chosen to no longer make love. They may even have accepted that in their relationship sex is something of the past. They've adjusted their life to its absence. We find that situation very unfortunate because, with more understanding, two people who have been together for some time and still love each other can easily find new ways of making love that include feelings of deeper vulnerability. It may not be as "sexual" or as hot as before, but it can be even more nourishing. In this chapter, we would like to bring some understanding for how it's possible to make love in a new way, a way which allows all your fears and insecurities to be present.

1. Validating Your Vulnerability

The first element is validating your vulnerability. Once you've decided to stop compensating or at least to become aware of your compensations, you're creating space to feel and accept your fears and insecurities. This includes understanding that your dysfunctions are symptoms of fears and insecurities. It takes courage to validate this part of you because there may be pressures from many sides to deny it, judge it or push it down. Sometimes a person will share with us that they can't accept their difficulties and fears in lovemaking because his or her partner doesn't like it. But when you yourself are not accepting your fears, you can't expect that your partner will. For instance, one woman told us that there is no space for her to accept her fears because her husband doesn't understand them and gets impatient with her. We tried to help her see that the problem was not with him but with her own lack of acceptance and judgment of her fears.

Harold, a sensitive man in his early forties, shared with us that he was disturbed because he was deeply in love with the woman he was with but compulsively distanced himself from her. This was especially strong in lovemaking. When they made love, he noticed that he would space out. She complained to him about this behavior and finally told him that unless something changed, she would leave him. When we explored this situation with him, it turned out that his distancing behavior came up most dramatically when they were making passionate love. He insisted that he made love this way because that is what she wanted. But eventually he confessed that he was afraid of not living up to her expectations. He wanted to pretend that he was a fully potent man. Underneath, he could feel that women terrified him.

There are strong internal voices that make it challenging for you to validate and accept your insecurities in sex. Voices such as:

- "You are making a big deal about nothing!"
- "Get on with it, move your energy!"
- "What is the matter with you?"
- "What are you so afraid of?"
- "You are just making up excuses to run away!"
- "You are a coward!
- "You are a terrible lover!"
- "You are just afraid of coming close to someone!"

- "You are using your past as an excuse!"

Perhaps from watching movies or reading, you have a concept of what perfect sex is, or you have listened to other people tell about their "fantastic" sexual experiences. When you're in shame, you compare yourself or push yourself with ideas of "better" sex. None of this helps you to be present to what is.

We have a client who is continually chasing after the perfect sexual experience. It is almost a religion for him. He is not in an intimate relationship with anyone and is quite disconnected from his vulnerability. This idea of the perfect sexual experience drives him and gives him purpose in life. He is perplexed why he doesn't have intimacy in his life. When you have ideas and expectations on yourself, you also have them on your partner and this creates tension and damages trust. Validating your vulnerability, your fears and insecurities, means being loving and accepting with whatever comes up — for both of you.

Sigmund, a man in his late forties, shared with us that he has been in love with a woman for six months and it was the best relationship he has ever had. Because he was so much in love, he also admitted that he feels more vulnerable than he has felt before. He's deeply troubled because his "erections are not as hard and as reliable as before." We pointed out to him that precisely because he is so in love with this woman, he is more susceptible to shock and dysfunction. He is probably beginning to touch places inside which are frightening and unfamiliar, and this brings up his insecurity. His vulnerability with this new woman is opening him up and taking away his usual compensations and protections. He doesn't mind the vulnerability but he is not at all happy that it is affecting his sexual prowess. In his mind, he cannot understand how a woman would want to stay with him if he is not "hard as a rock."

To validate your dysfunctions as symptoms of fear and insecurity, you also have to find a new basis for love. If you still believe that love is built on sexual performance, you will not be able allow space for fear and insecurity to come up. Sigmund was able to have "trouble free" sex until he fell more deeply in love. Now, he is being forced to look at deeper layers of his being which he denied earlier.

Validating your vulnerability also means embracing a dysfunction or fear even if you don't know where it comes from. Regina shared that while making love. Her vagina was contracted and her boyfriend was accusing her of wanting to castrate him. She could not understand why this was happening and felt utterly ashamed and discouraged. She even thought that maybe her boyfriend was right, that she was secretly trying to castrate him.

We explained to her that the muscle tightness in her vagina was a symptom of fear and mistrust. It relieved her to know this, but she had no memory of any sexual abuse. We explained to her that it was more important for her to validate the fear than it was to worry about the origin of the fear. Fear showing itself in the vagina does not necessarily mean that there has been a sexual trauma. It simply means that for whatever reason, you are not feeling safe at this moment. Regina still felt that her body reaction was excessive, and she wanted to open to her boyfriend more quickly. The pressure only made matters worse because she was invalidating her vulnerability.

2. Feeling and Listening to the Body

Once you begin to validate your sensitivity, you become more open to paying attention when this vulnerability shows itself. The easiest way, in our experience, is to learn to feel and listen to the body. This is the second element of opening to your vulnerability. Your body is exquisitely sensitive, but when you are lost in excitement or trying desperately to satisfy a sexual agenda, you don't listen.

To feel and listen to the body, you may need to slow things down. Fear and insecurity can be subtle and it can come very quickly, especially when you are making love. One moment you are feeling safe and open and the next, you suddenly feel frozen or deep in shame. You may not be aware of the frozenness or shame, but you may have thoughts in the mind covering what is happening in the body. One moment, all is going as you would like, and the next moment, you want to hide and be alone. Or suddenly you may find yourself judging your partner. You may not even know why your emotions or your body changed. It can be a sudden movement from your partner, a look or the way you are touched that triggers your reaction. Unless you slow things down, you can easily miss the point when the fear or insecurity arise and compensate either by speeding up or disconnecting and dissociating. You may continue making love but you are no longer present.

Here are some sensations to look for:

- Constriction, pain, tightness, numbness, or emptiness in the genitals.
- Constriction, shallow breathing, trembling or an emptiness and hollowness in the chest.
- The heart rate speeding up.
- Hot or cold sensations in your body and in your extremities,
- Tightness in other parts of your body – the neck, back or stomach or belly.
- Feeling restless or tired
- Feeling uncomfortable

3. Speaking It Out

a. Sharing Your Sexual Shame and Secrets

Sometimes you have so much shame about something connected to your sexuality that you hide it even from your intimate partner. Perhaps it is a family secret, a fantasy, a dysfunction or a perversion. By hiding it, it eats away at you and disturbs the intimacy you share with your partner. When you risk speaking out and sharing what you are ashamed of and have hidden, it is very empowering. By sharing, not only do you unload what you have been holding inside, you also discover that others also have secrets that they have hidden.

Sometimes it is painful when you take the risk to share your sexual shame and secrets. One woman told her boyfriend that she had a sexual trauma and needed for him to be slow when they made love. He responded by telling her that he was sick of this "wounded child stuff" and didn't want to hear it. In such a case, risking exposing your vulnerability may help you to realize that you are in a relationship which is no longer nourishing because it is not safe to be vulnerable. There is never any guarantee that you will get the reception you want when you open up these delicate topics, but in our experience, it is worth the risk.

When you share, you also begin to see connections between past traumas and your life and sexuality today. Rachel shared in a group that for many years she was having severe problems with her digestion. She felt that she needed to talk about this because she was so ashamed. As we asked her questions, she confessed that her father had abused her sexually. She had no idea that these two – her health problems and her abuse — were related. But as she continued to talk about herself, she could feel how unsafe she felt inside and how she had minimized her abuse without feeling how it affected her body and her life.

Speaking out also includes revealing a specific shame, perhaps about your body or about your sexuality in general. One man shared with us that when he confessed to his partner that he was ashamed that his erection was not hard enough, she said that she didn't like it when his penis was too hard because she felt it was much more loving and sensitive when it was softer. Another man told us that he started taking Viagra without telling his wife. But when they were making love, she felt something different and was puzzled. When he admitted that he had taken the pill, she was upset that he hadn't told her because she could feel that he was more compensated and less present. The more vulnerable we allow ourselves to be, the more present we become and whatever we hold back affects our ability to be present.

b. Sharing About Your Sexual Abuse

It's our experience that if you are in an intimate relationship, it is essential that your lover knows if you have experienced sexual trauma in the past. We also feel that it is important that both people learn and understand what it means for lovemaking. Otherwise, you might minimize the effects this has on your life and your sexuality today. Angela was sexually abused by her father and was anorexic as a teenager. Her mother not only did not protect her from her father's sexual attentions but also minimized her fears and insecurities all her childhood. Now, as an adult, she finds that she pushes her husband away sexually as well as emotionally and sometimes attacks him for no apparent reason. When she first came to work with us, she said that she felt that her "wounded child" was over-indulgent and she exaggerated her trauma. With time, she could begin to appreciate how shocked she is and how terrified she feels of letting anyone, especially a man, come close.

> *We want to emphasize that the details of our abuse story are not the most important part of our healing and of our returning to healthy and nourishing sexuality. Often the facts of our trauma are confusing and unclear and we may never know what happened. Sometimes we may embellish on what actually happened or even change or confuse the persons involved. To fixate on proving to ourselves or to someone else what actually happened can be a distraction. What matters is to validate that, in some basic way, we have been traumatized and our sexuality today suffers from this trauma. And when we are sharing our abuse, this is what is most important.*

Often, you may be exposing your fears and insecurities without having a clue about where they come from. But when your sexuality is disturbed, there is a reason. You may not know the reason, but unless you understand that your fear and insecurity is a result of some kind of past trauma, you may easily blame yourself and feel deep shame and guilt. You may never know where your fear and shock comes from. It is enough simply to connect the dysfunction, the body symptoms, the insecurities and the fears to the *fact* of feeling unsafe or invaded in some way in the past.

c. What About Fantasies and Sex Tools?

When it comes to sharing about sexual perversions and fantasies, we enter into a delicate and sensitive area. Honestly, we are not supportive of using fantasies, sex tools, orgies or threesomes to add "spice" to your sexuality. And the reason is that it can easily lead to "objective sex." Fantasies and devices are often symptoms of either repressed sexuality, insecurities about yourself as a person, or unresolved interpersonal conflicts.

But in our experience, it is important to share them because if you don't, it can create distance between you and your partner, dishonesty, guilt and mistrust. However, hiding your fantasies or voicing them *without exploring what is behind them* can be damaging to a relationship. If you recognize that all of this can be a cover for shame and fear, it can increase your intimacy by making you more vulnerable.

A man shared with us that he secretly and regularly rented pornographic videos or watched it on the Internet. When he finally found the courage to tell his partner about this, she was upset. She was happy that he had shared it but she was not happy with his continuing the behavior. He was willing to admit to himself and to her that it was an addiction and to seek help for it.

Another man we worked with wanted to make love with bondage. He was afraid to admit it but when he shared it with his partner, she was happy that he admitted it because she could feel it anyway. He also wanted her to participate with him in this kind of lovemaking. He claimed it helped "turn him on" and "feel like a man," and for him it was a perfectly legitimate way of making love. She was not interested, and they fought about it. Fortunately, he was willing to go deeper and work with the shame and insecurity that was underneath and eventually to see that in this way he was compensating.

A young man in his twenties shared with us that he was always fantasizing about making love to many women even though he was in love with the woman he was with. He felt guilty about it and she could also feel that he was withholding something. He had fantasies of having orgies with many women, taking women from behind and enjoying their screams of pleasure when he made them reach orgasm. Without invalidating or judging his fantasies, we helped him to go the roots of his insecurity and shame. They didn't disappear, but we suggested that rather than give energy to them or take steps to act them out, he could continue to explore and feel his fears of opening and becoming more vulnerable with his partner.

It is your choice what you decide to give your attention to. If you sincerely believe that acting out fantasies will make you more fulfilled sexually, then it could a good idea to investigate for yourself if this is true. And if you feel that fantasies enhances your closeness with your partner that is another idea that can be worth investigating. Find out for yourself. It's our experience that in the end, they neither enhance sexual fulfillment or intimacy. But we never want people to do anything from an idea that it might "better" to behave a certain way. We would like people to find out for themselves what works for them. All we do is share our own experience as a long-term couple.

In our experiences, fantasies, violent sex and sex games keep sexuality objective and it is a cover for shame and fears of closeness. One man shared with us that he was not interested in having deep, intimate sex with his partner. He just wanted to be sexy, feel sexy, and to have sex that was hot and hard. He admitted that this was objectifying his woman and when he made love, he was thinking of just "fucking women." His girlfriend appreciated his being so direct and it was a relief for her when he was so honest. She added that she could enjoy making love in this way as long as he stayed sensitive and respected her limits. But as he explored more deeply, he could see that this approach to sex was a cover for deep insecurities about himself as a man. He was out of work, without money and feeling insecure about himself as a man in the world.

d. Sharing Your Needs

Finally, speaking out also includes talking about what you need when you are making love. This is also a delicate topic because expressing needs can easily become confused with expressing demands. Expressing needs can come from your vulnerability and can make the other person feel closer to you. Expressing demands comes from your protection; it's a power game and pushes the person away.

For some of us, it's terrifying to say what we need. There may be so much fear that the other person, even if it is your intimate partner, will not accept it. They may feel controlled, not listen, get angry, or minimize what you say and reject you. There can be much shame, especially if you are touching fears while making love that you have not encountered before. It can also bring up shame to talk about what you would like in lovemaking and what you need to help you open. You may have a strong conditioning that it's not okay to talk about your sexuality or that your partner should "just know" what you need and like without your having to say anything.

All of the aspects of sharing vulnerability about your sexuality that we have been describing can be extremely challenging. There is no telling if the relationship can survive the test of vulnerability and opening your sexual vulnerability to your partner is one of the biggest tests. If you don't take this step, the consequences can be extreme. You can stop making love, you can become resentful of your partner, you can compensate in your sexuality just to please your partner and betray your own body, or you can hide your shame and fears inside pretending that they are not there.

However, when you take this step to open and share yourself honestly, it can become profoundly nourishing both for yourself and for the intimacy. You are touching places inside that need to be opened and shared and to do so brings deep compassion, self-respect and prepares the ground for much deeper love and trust.

Keys For Sharing Your Vulnerability in Sex

1. Validate Your Vulnerability Rather Than Minimizing, Denying or Judging Your Fears and Insecurities.
2. Take Time to Feel and Share Fears and Insecurity As They Show Themselves In The Body. This Includes Feeling and Sharing the Fear Behind Dysfunctions, Dissociating or Wanting to Pull Away and Avoid Sexual Contact.
3. Share Your Vulnerability — Share Your Shame Around Sex, Share Your Sexual Abuse, Share Your Fantasies and the Fear and Shame Underneath.
4. Share What You Need in Sex to Help You to Open, Feel Safe and Relaxed.

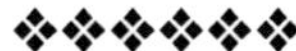

Chapter 10
"How Can I Keep My Love Alive?" Honoring the Flower of Love

Sex is easier than love. Many people confuse sex for love because in the passion of sex, we can feel "in love" — taken over by the intensity of the connection and the sex. These experiences are wonderful, but they are not love. In these experiences, it is as though existence is giving you a little taste to motivate you to take the deeper and more arduous journey of discovering love. Unless you undertake this journey, you might easily get bitter and disappointed, and blame your partner when the taste is gone.

> *Love means placing our most delicate flower in the hands of another person who, in some ways, will always be a stranger. To love one another, we have to be willing to take and nourish each other's flower as if it were the most precious offering in the world. Our ability to love someone tests our level of maturity. It challenges us to become deeper, more aware, more sensitive, more loving and more compassionate.*

Your regressed child acts out. And often when it does, it threatens the delicate fabric of love. You cannot pretend that this part of you doesn't exist simply because you would like to be more mature, less selfish, reactive or mistrustful or needy. In deep intimacy with another person, there are times when you will be insensitive or perhaps abusive (humiliating, neglecting, irritable, manipulative, disparaging, ignoring, unsupportive, raging or perhaps even verbally or physically abusive) toward your partner. You can repair anything if you are willing to feel the effect of your action or mood and sincerely and profoundly honor the love and your partner's sensitivity. If you can feel your partner's hurt and take responsibility for your behavior, you can heal the hurt and even get closer. It all depends on how much you value the love you are creating and realize how exquisitely fragile it is.

In this chapter, we are going to discuss what we have discovered are the basic ingredients for nourishing the delicate flower of love.

Learning What Damages Love and Trust

1. "Open Relationships?"

Sometimes we say in our work, in reference to love relationships, that we have a choice. We can choose superficial or even extended love stories, but stories where we are not truly open and vulnerable. We hide our fears of opening and loving deeply behind power games, control and codependency. Or, we can risk opening deeply to another person in an equal, committed and long-term relationship. Even the thought of losing this person is terrifying. We know that one day, because we are mortal beings, we will lose this person. We also know that this loss will be shattering, but we will also recover and go on anyway.

People often ask us for our opinion about affairs — more specifically, how to deal with the desire to have an affair or the fact that they or their partner have had one or are having one. Each situation is different, and sometimes it might be the right move to have an affair or to decide to have short love stories rather than be in a committed relationship. But we do tell people to take responsibility for their choices.

Affairs have an attraction. There is a part of you who likes variety, and when you have been with someone for a while, it is natural to long for a change. There is the thrill of attraction and conquest, it might be free of emotional complications and perhaps, and you are rekindling the sexual excitement that you have been missing. Sometimes having an affair may be the right thing because it can wake you up to the fact that the love with your partner has died and you need either to do everything you can to revive it or to let it go.

For example, we were working with a woman who is married and has three young children. She admitted to us that she was having an affair. She had told her husband that she was seeing someone but did not reveal the whole truth — that she was in love and making love to this person.

"How is your relationships with your husband?" we asked

"I love him very much and I love having a family with him, but I am more his mother than his lover. We make love and I enjoy it but with this other person. I feel met in a way that I have never been met before."

"Do you feel that it is a conflict for you to be with both?" we asked.

"For now, it feels okay. I don't think he could handle it if I told him the whole truth and I don't want to do that. I am so happy with this new person, I can't even tell you. And I don't want to have to choose."

We supported her to continue with the affair, as it was obviously very important for her. She had never been in a relationship where she was not in control. Her pattern of being the mother was a war game in disguise because it kept her securely in control. In her old relationship, she was acting out an old and familiar pattern and this had killed the energy and the sexuality. With this new person, she was not in control, and she could experience how nourishing it was to be an equal. Their sexuality was on fire. However, the situation of juggling two lovers was unstable and sooner or later would have to change. She would have to meet and cross that bridge when she came to it.

And sure enough, shortly after, she did have to make a decision. Her husband discovered the whole truth of her affair and gave her an ultimatum. "Either drop the affair or leave." She did the former but was miserable and longed to see her new partner. When we last spoke with her, she said she that nothing much had improved with her husband even though she was not betraying him anymore. She was still not really facing the crossroad honestly. Choosing to stay with her husband meant recognizing her controls and opening to him more deeply. Choosing to leave meant facing the fears of leaving the family and the security it brought her.

In our experience, when you create an affair, it is a sign that something is going on in the relationship that needs to be looked at and dealt with. You may hope to maintain both relationships and even keep it a secret for a while, but eventually the secret usually comes out one way or another. And even in the meantime, this situation takes a huge toll of the trust and the intimacy.

A few years ago, a woman who was doing our training became disturbed with us because we were teaching that, in our opinion, "open relationships" don't work. By open relationships, we mean having other lovers and at the same time hoping to preserve or deepen intimacy in the "primary" relationship. By "don't work" we mean that sooner or later, in our experience, the relationship self-destructs. She claimed that although her boyfriend had other lovers, they were fine together. It kept things more alive, she said. It kept them from taking each other for granted and it kept their sex more "juicy."

In our experience, love is too delicate and our vulnerability too fragile to sustain the kind of connection where one or both partners make love to others. To open and share yourself intimately with another person is such a delicate phenomenon that when you make love to others it damages the delicate fabric of trust that takes years to develop and grow. By the second week of the training, six months later, she was no longer so sure she wanted things to stay the same with her boyfriend. By the third week, after nine months, they had broken up.

It is not uncommon for couples to have affairs, but the question is if a relationship can recover from an affair. It depends. The trust can be repaired if the love is deep enough and if you are willing to feel the pain you have caused. And your partner needs to feel that you sincerely feel that pain. To recover the trust and the love, you also need to find out what it was that attracted you to have an affair and to get to the root of this issue with your partner. You may need professional help to work it through.

A man was in pain because his girlfriend had had an affair. Whenever he brought up his pain about what had happened, her response was that he was "just being a victim and it was time for him to get over it."

"It is not such a big deal," she said. "Anyway, it is my freedom to make love to whomever I want and you just have to handle it yourself if you get jealous. Also, I get bored with you when you are too needy."

They stayed together, albeit not very harmoniously, and a year later, he had an affair. Now it was her turn to become jealous and in pain. But at least she was able to understand what he had felt earlier. And at this point, it was possible for us to work with them to repair the trust because they could both feel how painful it is to damage the trust.

2. Dishonesty

We are all human, and most of us are not totally honest with ourselves — let alone our most intimate partners. But there are degrees of dishonesty. Some of your dishonesties may be relatively harmless. But other kinds of dishonesties create distance between you and the one you love. It slowly erodes the trust. Dishonesty comes from fear and sometimes the fear is so great that you cannot find the courage to tell the truth. Unfortunately, it can become a habit to be dishonest.

One client of ours was chronically dishonest. She would habitually make promises to those close to her but invariably would not live up to her word. It was similar in relation to us. She would make a commitment and then break it. And it happened so often that we slowly stopped believing in anything she said. Others who knew her told us the same thing — that they could no longer trust anything she said. This is a painful way to live.

A client who was having an affair told us that she was too afraid to tell her husband "because she didn't want to hurt him." When she went to spend nights or weekends with her lover, she would find different kinds of excuses to explain her absence to her husband and pack in secret so that he wouldn't suspect anything. She was convinced that he didn't know about the affair, but noticed that he had become increasingly moody, childish and sexually needy. We explained to her that even if he didn't know consciously what she was up to, somewhere inside he knew it even if he didn't know that he knew it. This was what was causing him to become disturbed, needy, moody, regressed and demanding.

You pay a heavy price for dishonesty when it concerns something so vital as an affair or another person's being able to count on your living up to what you say. It is a betrayal to the other person, a betrayal to yourself and a betrayal of the love between you. You may have too much fear inside to find the courage to be honest but still, it is important to feel the damage that you are causing.

3. Violence in Any Form

A couple came to see us because the man had frequent rage attacks and once had hit his partner. He had apologized for his behavior, but she no longer felt safe. He claimed that most of the time he just shouted and occasionally hit a wall, and only once had he lost control and actually hit her. He realized that by hitting her, he had crossed the line and sincerely felt bad about it. But he felt provoked because he claimed she was so demanding and hysterical. In his mind, he was doing well by containing his rage and only shouting or taking it out on walls and doors. What he did not realize was that his rage attacks were terrorizing her.

When we asked her about her behavior, she admitted that often she nagged him, and it was true that she was demanding and hard on him at times. We explained that both of them were violating each other — his violation was physical abuse and hers was emotional. They could see how they were being disrespectful to each other. He promised to take more responsibility for his anger and frustration by working with his own aggression in a safe place and making efforts not to act out his rage in front of her. She agreed to find new ways to talk to him when she was stressed and take more responsibility for her demanding behavior.

> *We are often unaware of how our behavior impacts our partner. Sometimes our behavior is much more violent that we realize. But we are not in touch with the violence because we are not feeling what our partner feels. The behavior can be blatant or it can be subtle. Either way, it can be extremely damaging to the love we are trying to nourish and deepen.*

4. Trying to Change Each Other

In a long-term relationship one of the most significant questions you can ask yourself is, "Can I love and accept this person even if he or she doesn't change?" People change but not according to your expectations. If you're waiting for them to change, you will suffer and the relationship will suffer. This, in our experience, is perhaps the single most challenging hurdle for deepening love. In a short-term affair, you can be satisfied with only taking in and accepting the parts of the other person that you like. Not so with love. Love is more exacting. It requires taking in the whole person, including his or her fears and insecurities, defenses and protective behaviors.

> *Learning to love involves trying to understand the other person — learning how and why he or she feels, think and behaves. It means taking the vulnerability of the other person into your heart.*

Anders was pushing his girlfriend Brigitte away with his aggressive pressure and criticism. He would get upset when he felt that she was not being present with him, and he would berate her when he felt that she was not setting adequate limits on her teenage daughter. When he started working with us, we helped him to understand that all his insistence that she change was a way of avoiding to feel his own abandonment wound. He understood intellectually but it didn't change his behavior. Finally, she had had enough of the way he was treating her and she left him.

Her leaving plunged him into a deep despair, but he was willing to feel his pain and continue working with us. We guided him to learn how to contain his pain, frustration and anger by going in whenever he was provoked, feeling his body and gently breathing into the places where he felt the disturbance. As he practiced this simple technique, it became easier for him. At one point, he understood from his belly that the way he had been treating her was not only disrespectful but also an avoidance of himself.

Bringing the Focus Back to Yourself

We often say in our work that intention is everything. Your intention frequently determines the outcome of any endeavor you go into. In a relationship, if your intention is to learn about yourself rather than to use the other person as a way of avoiding yourself, you are on the right track from the beginning. Many of us may have been conditioned with romantic fantasies that the right relationship is meant to make us happy and shelter us from fear, loneliness and insecurity. Wrong intention. You might even believe that if your relationship is not providing that, there is something fatally wrong with it. It is a painful and destructive misunderstanding.

As long as you stay focused on how your partner needs to change, on their deficiencies, on how he or she needs to be there for you, you don't look at yourself. Every moment of disappointment and frustration is a moment to look inside. In those moments, the automatic habit, even the compulsion, is to look to the other person. But these are the times when a sincere willingness to take the focus off the other and bring it back to yourself can make the difference between sabotaging or deepening love. It is helpful to know your own trauma story enough to know how and why you get triggered and how you habitually react. But it is even more helpful to find the inner space to contain the frustration. And that is not easy.

Learning to love involves a maturing and a giving. It helps to realize from the outset that love is not about getting what we want but learning to give more and more and a willingness to accept frequent frustration and disappointments.

We were recently giving a session to a couple who fought whenever they made love — or *tried* to make love. She felt invaded whenever she sensed that he wanted something from her, including his desire and expectation to ejaculate. Although she had no memories of earlier sexual trauma, it was clear that she was supersensitive to feeling invaded and did not trust her ability to set limits. As a result, she avoided making love altogether. This, in turn, made him feel rejected and increased his agitation and desire. We suggested that they try making love in a way where orgasm is not the goal. We also attempted to make him understand that unless he could help her to feel safe when they made love, she could never relax and would not be open to making love. It was a true challenge for him to focus just on giving and set aside his preoccupation with receiving. We encouraged her to share her fears with him openly, realizing that they are deeper and older than the present moment when they are making love, rather than blame him as the cause of her fear and feelings of being unsafe.

Another client of ours decided that he was finished with relationship. "I just want to put my energy into other areas," he told us. However, what he could not yet see was that he was driving women away because whenever he gets close to someone, he blamed them whenever they didn't behave as he wanted them to. We have known this person for some years and notice that in all his intimate relationships — man or woman — he is a compulsive blamer. Rather than look at himself and what underlies the reactions he gets from others, he blames. He's still not able to ask himself the correct question, "rather than making others wrong, what is it that I need to learn about myself in these situations — what I have done that pushes people away?"

Taking In The Whole Person

It is easy to love yourself when you are in your essence and your beauty is being seen and felt, your energy flows, and you are feeling at home in yourself. The challenge comes when you are not in this essence layer.

> *The challenge and the growth is not to love ourselves when we are in our essence, but to accept and love ourselves when we are in protection or when we are in the wounded layer feeling lonely, insecure, afraid or full of shame.*

The paradox is that the moment you fully accept whatever is happening, even if it is the *woundedness* or the protection, it becomes part of the essence. This is the beauty and the magic of life, almost like having found the magic key that unlocks the doors to the treasure chest. When you fight, judge and want your protection or wounds to go away, they only get stronger and deeper. The way through is to truly bring love and compassion to yourself in these difficult or painful moments.

It is the same when it comes to loving another. Their essence is easy to love but it is hard to love their protection and wounds. When you come close to another person, you are usually attracted by some aspect of their essence. It's not difficult to love someone when they are with themselves, "in their energy," alive, responsive, open, communicative, sensitive, sexually available, adventurous and free, insightful, loving, attentive, strong, self-assured — or some combination of these qualities. But it is not so easy to take someone in when they are fearful and insecure, especially if the fears and insecurities cause them to hold back, become withdrawn, angry and manipulative or addictive. It is even harder when he or she denies all of this and claims to be "alive and with an open heart."

> *Learning to love involves getting to know and accept all of the three layers of ourselves and our partner. It means recognizing and accepting when we*

or our partner is in protection or in fear and shame. And to do that, it helps to know our story as well as our partner's story.

The past is not significant in itself. The past is over. And if it were just the past, then it would be merely an interesting curiosity. But when it affects who you are and how you live and behave today, it is more than a curiosity. It brings deep understanding and compassion to yourself and the one you love when you understand this intimately.

The shame or trauma story includes:

- How you were repressed in your life energies – your sexuality, power, feelings, joy, creativity and intuition.
- What your childhood environment was, how you were received into the world, who nurtured you and how you were nurtured.
- How much stress your caretakers were under, what stresses you received as neglect, abuse, and lack of support, pressure, criticism and judgments.
- The roles that you were conditioned to play such as a caretaker or emotional support for a parent, living the unfulfilled dreams of your parents, or being compared to a sibling or role model.

All of these situations are ripe for creating shame and trauma and, most likely, you and your partner still carry the scars. The scars determine how you will react today to stress, what triggers your fears of abandonment or insecurity and what makes you feel overwhelmed, unloved and disrespected.

You can uncover much of this about yourself as you do work with yourself. But for the flowering of love, you also need to do know, feel and understand the trauma story of your partner and take it into your heart. The ways that you trigger each other and the ways that you respond to these triggers is no great mystery. The clues are all revealed in your shame and trauma story. When you can anticipate your partner's sensitivities, you can also take care not to throw salt in their open wounds. This does not mean that you have to repress your energy or be careful in the sense of not being true to yourself, but it is more about a deep sensitivity to the other person you love. As you mature, you naturally become more respectful of the other person. As you learn to honor your own needs and learn not to betray yourself or your body, you become less obsessed and fixated on getting your needs met and more able to be flexible and understanding.

A couple in a workshop shared that they were quarreling much of the time. He was upset because she was pushing him away. She complained that he was not sensitive to her and did things that irritated her such as making too much noise around the house, and being too "needy." They benefited from learning about each other's story. He was given away by his biological parents to an orphanage and was raised for the first seven years of his life by punitive and abusive nuns. Then, he was sent to a foster home where his foster parents were not abusive, gave him much freedom, but little closeness.

His wife could not remember much about her childhood earlier than age twelve. But she did know that her parents fought a lot and she suspected that her father was attracted to her sexually. And as a teenager, he had made abusive comments to her about her sexuality. As they unraveled and shared their stories with each other it became easier to take each other into their hearts. He began to understand that when she pushed him away, she was really afraid of being abused and not being seen, and he could then approach her in a new way that enabled her to open to him.

She understood that his making noise and being "needy" was his attempt to get her attention. His old trauma of being unwanted was being rekindled through their love and all that was needed was for her to acknowledge him and make him feel wanted. Through this kind of understanding and love something begins to relax in both partners and the old wounds slowly heal.

A delicate question is, what you should accept in your partner? Do you accept their addictive behavior or their aggression? Recently we worked with a woman who shared that her boyfriend was addicted to marijuana and had no motivation to quit in spite of her objections. He could see no problem with his smoking and minimized her complaints that it made him not present. Furthermore, he was aggressive and insensitive with her in other ways and when she complained about this behavior, he told her that it was her problem that she was so "oversensitive." In the course of the workshop, it became increasingly clear to her that she was in a dysfunctional relationship that was a re-enactment (and re-traumatizing) of her shame and feelings of being abandoned by her father. It became clear that it was not healthy for her to remain in this relationship, and she awaited the time when she found the courage to leave him.

We often work with couples where one is addicted to a substance such as marijuana or alcohol, or to some behavior such as watching pornography or having frequent affairs. It is a serious problem because the addiction serves as another lover, one who is often more reliable and predictable. It is difficult for the love to flourish between two people while this is occurring. Every situation is different, but we stress that when there is a problem of this kind, it needs to be addressed or the relationship will eventually die.

Taking in the other person also does not include accepting disrespect, invasion or abuse. In such situations, you're called upon, for your own growth and self-respect, to learn to set limits. Your partner's trauma story and his or her sensitivities may explain abusive or insensitive and disrespectful behavior, *but it does not excuse it.* If you don't learn to stand up for yourself when your boundaries and self-respect is being abused, you take on the role of a victim. That role is not healthy. In setting limits, you are not saying "no!" to the whole person; you are simply saying "no!" to disrespectful behavior. However, if you find yourself in a situation where your limits are not being honored even when you affirm them, then it might be time to say "no!" *and* "goodbye!"

Making Time For Love

All too often, in the frantic pace of our life, you don't take the time to love each other and to connect to each other. Everything else becomes more important. You find yourself becoming stressed and overly involved in the practical details of life, and lovemaking and closeness start to fall away. You might even feel that you are missing your partner, but you are so stressed and your mind is so busy with practical things that sex or even connecting seems like the last thing you want to do. Or you may try to use sex to relieve stress which is not such a good idea. Also, men tend want to do that more than women, who generally find that kind of sex not so attractive. The flower of love needs water and nourishment. Also, when you don't take time to come back to the body, you forget about it. Your energy goes into the head and then you don't feel anything below the waist or even in the heart.

A man was sharing that he was upset because he felt that his wife didn't seem to have enough time for him. He said that he was quite self-reliant and enjoyed spending time alone, but when too much time went by without love making, he began to feel deprived and then would become irritable, withdrawn and moody. We knew from previous work with him that he was in a healthy and loving relationship with his partner and that their problem was not coming from unresolved interpersonal dynamics or lack of sexual interest. It seemed to simply be a matter of time and priority.

His wife was deeply involved in her artwork, and because it was so absorbing and nourishing for her she could easily get lost in it and forget to connect with him. Then at night she was so exhausted that they would watch TV and go to sleep. And this had become a routine. We helped him to see that part of his feelings of deprivation were coming from his abandonment wound, but we also suggested that he invite his wife for a date and make this a regular occurrence. At first, he was reluctant because he wanted it to be spontaneous, and also he wanted her to come to him. Furthermore, he wasn't sure she would agree. We invited him to set his pride and fear aside and go for it anyway. He found, to his surprise, that his partner was very willing to agree to this new solution because she also missed him and their physical intimacy and appreciated the encouragement to get away from her art. They set up biweekly appointments to spend an hour in the afternoon in bed and he discovered that he felt much less deprived.

In our work, we find that this situation is quite common. Couples let time go by, getting so involved in the practicalities and stresses of the daily routine of their lives, that they forget about intimacy and lovemaking. And when you let time slip by without loving each other and without putting your bodies together to connect, you get "out of the mood." People often tell us that even though they feel deep love for their partner, they just don't "feel sexual" anymore. We have explored in previous chapters that this problem can have many causes, but sometimes it can be as simple as disciplining yourself a little to get out of the mind and back into your bodies, to set aside the stuff of your daily life and make time for loving.

Many of us may have the idea that sex has to be spontaneous and we both have to feel turned on before making love. This may be true for "level one sex" and for people who are newly together. But long-term couples often need to make it a point to remember to make love. You may not be in the mood simply because you have allowed your energy to get lost in practicalities. Life is short and love is precious. It is a shame to let time slip by obsessed with practicalities and forget about watering the flower of love.

Practical matters have a tendency to pull you to take care of them, but the list can be endless. Many things can wait. Unless you set a time aside that suits both of you, it may not happen. Another helpful approach is making a point of taking regular holidays away from all the distractions of home. It is wonderful to be able to take a week in some romantic and beautiful setting, but sometimes just a night or two at a hotel can be enough to remind you to make love.

There are ways to make time for love other than actually making love. It is also important for deepening love to find common interests and share time and activities together. When you spend time together, you are communicating on a non-verbal level that nourishes the love in deep ways. And just as you may need to use a little discipline and intention to remember to make love, you also may need to do the same when finding things to share. When you love someone deeply, it feels natural to tune into each other and step into each other's worlds.

For instance, Amana loves to watch the Oprah Show. At first I was like, "give me a break! No way am I going to watch a show with women screaming at celebrities and dealing with topics like weight loss and the latest fashions and interior design." So when Oprah time came up, I would sweetly hand her the headphones. But either Oprah changed or I changed because I have become a total Oprah fan. Some of her shows are so profound and penetrating that we even record them for our work.

Love thrives when you realize that it takes a continual willingness to nurture it and to keep it fresh by making it an opportunity to learn and grow together. Every situation and every relationship is different. Sometimes, because of irreconcilable differences and lack of communication, it may be time to move on. But when you realize that love requires commitment, perseverance, understanding and a willingness to go through hard times, your need to move on diminishes and if you do decide to go, you do it for the right reasons.

Keys for Nourishing the Flower of Love

1. Learning What Damages Trust and Love

    a. "Open Relationships"

    b. Dishonesty

    c. Disrespect and Violence of Any Kind

    d. Attempting to Change the Other Person

2. Bringing Back the Focus Onto Yourself and Taking Responsibility (Rather than Casting Blame on Our Partner) and Identifying Your Patterns and Working On Yourself

3. Taking In the Whole Person – Learning to Accept Your Partner With All His or Her Fears, Insecurities and Defense

4. Making Time For Love — Creating Time Away from Practicalities to Connect and Make Love

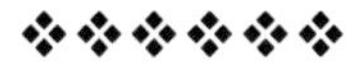

Chapter 11
"My Relationship is Not Going to Make Me Whole."
Letting Go of the Illusions of Love

In our experience, many of the problems of relating don't come from interpersonal difficulties. They arise because one or both people are not happy in their life and with themselves. A relationship suffers when you count on it to make you happy or when you count on the other person to take away your anxiety, pain and loneliness. Then you take your frustrations out on your partner when life is not as you would like it to be or when you're not feeling at ease with yourself. By making the other person responsible for your pain, you pave the way for endless power struggles. Both people feel wronged, disappointed and disillusioned.

Your Lack of Fulfillment Can Sabotage Love

Recently, we were working with a couple who came to us because they were, in their own words, "fighting all the time." Their sexuality was not a problem and both shared that they had never experienced lovemaking before which was so nourishing and relaxed. But he complained that she was controlling and rigid and "always had to have things her way." She was equally upset because she claimed that he would have frequent rage attacks and blame her for "the smallest things." As we delved deeper into their relating dynamics, we saw that the problem was not anything between them or in the way they were communicating but that he was not fulfilled in his life and was not living or expressing his creativity.

She was a successful businesswoman and he was out of work and undecided about what to do next. Because of this situation, he was unhappy with himself, resented her success and her enjoyment in her work, and also resented that she was paying the bills. Although there were minor issues between them that needed to be looked at, this was the primary cause of his anger and discontent and why they frequently had conflicts. We helped him to focus his energy on becoming more clear and directed in his life, even if it meant a physical separation for a while during education or training.

This issue of not feeling fulfilled in your life can also affect your sexuality. As an example, we were working with a couple who told us that although their relationship was going well, their sexuality was not. She felt that their sex was too hard for her and it caused her to back away. When we asked him how it was for him, he openly admitted that he was taking out his frustrations in sex because he wasn't happy in his work life. He was a graphic designer and currently having trouble finding work. He felt he was being paid too little for those jobs that he did get. He had difficulties believing in himself and easily compromised in the work place.

Later, he felt bitter and resentful that he had sold himself too cheaply for his work and this would fuel his rage. Without being aware of this dynamic and without having another way of working with his anger, he would then act it out in their lovemaking. We worked with his fears of setting limits and with his feeling of inadequacy. Through some very sincere work he was able to begin to take the risk to ask for a fee for his jobs that he felt comfortable with. This in turn created more self-respect. With that foundation, their lovemaking slowly changed.

When you come closer to someone, it's easy to forget or lose yourself. One of the issues which we deal with often with couples is their having become so enmeshed with each other that one or both have given up their own lives. And in the process, they lose their self-esteem. Then they often attempt to control each other's lives to the point of judging, advising, criticizing or even humiliating each other. For instance, in one case, a woman in a couple forbade her partner to watch television because she felt that it was bad for his spiritual development. (When we last spoke with her, she told us that she had not only become comfortable with his watching but had joined him and was having a good time.)

In another example, a man continually commented on his partner's eating habits because he felt that she was not eating healthy food. But he had to admit that he kept a tight rein on his own eating habits because he was so afraid of indulging and "losing it." And every so often, he *would* lose it. Sometimes, he found himself eating three desserts after dinner when he went to a restaurant. This kind of "negative symbiosis" occurs when you turn to the relationship to give you meaning in life at the expense of developing your own creativity and aliveness. It can also happen when you have lost touch with your inner sense of direction and then look to the other for guidance.

Developing Inner Space

Finding contentment in your life also includes finding ways to face your own fears rather than depending on your partner to shelter you from your fears, insecurities and anxieties. In our work, we use the word "inner space" to define the inner centeredness, in which we can find some detachment from the disturbances that arise. When you have not cultivated "inner space," you can easily expect to get it from your partner. You may even believe that this is one of the criteria of love.

Perhaps one of life's greatest lessons is to learn to face your own fears and insecurities, to notice when these get provoked in your daily life and to find ways to deal with your fears in healthy ways.

> *Often what creates conflict between partners has to do with the degree of stress that one or both are in. Contentment in our life strongly depends on finding ways to soothe our nervous system away*

from tension toward relaxation — ways that are not dependent on our partner.

We find it helpful when teaching this concept to imagine that your energy and your nervous system act like a barometer. The barometer is divided into three parts. On the left side is what we call "the relaxation zone," in the middle "the tension zone," and on the right, "the overwhelm zone" or "red zone". We would all love to live in the relaxation zone but, in fact, because of the normal stresses and pressures of everyday life mixed with our own inner pressures and expectations, we mostly live in the tension zone. When you get triggered by some outside or internal stress, your needle moves toward the right and can easily move into the overwhelm zone. When this happens, you naturally blame, rage or complain about whatever provoked you into feeling overwhelmed. But the problem is not the trigger — it is the state of your nervous tension. When you are more relaxed and at home within yourself, the same thing that might have caused a major disturbance may only cause a little ripple, if any at all.

It is also important to find ways to soothe yourself and your nervous system before you make love rather than coming to your partner with all of your unresolved tensions inside. Steve and Beatrice booked a couples session with us because they were having difficulties with sex. Steve began by saying, "She is always rejecting me. Nothing is ever good enough for her. She has to have the room right, the smells right, the energy just right. And now I am coming fast all the time, which never happened before with other women that I have been with."

Beatrice responded, "He comes home from work all tense and expects to make love. But I don't want to make love to him when he is like that. So naturally, I want to make things better so that I can open. I don't open very easily anyway, and when he is all angry and bothered by the situation at work, I can't open at all. And then he blames me for being closed."

We asked them what each of them could do to make the other person feel more relaxed and open.

Steve said, "I want to feel that you want me and aren't always rejecting me."

Beatrice said, "I want you! I really, *really* love you. But first I want you to relax."

We validated both of their fears and their concerns. We suggested that Steve do a meditation when he came home, a meditation that we had made, which included a half hour on intense dance music followed by fifteen minutes of guided silent meditation. We also suggested to Beatrice that she share her fears about lovemaking rather than making a habit of finding excuses in the environment to avoid sex.

> *Because we live mostly in the "tension zone," we also are easily impacted by the tension of our partner, especially as we become more and more symbiotic with each other something that naturally happens the longer we are with someone. We feel the tension and anxiety of the other person and it feels like our own. Then we may blame the other person for being "so uptight."*

Sandra and Alex have been a together for many years. They love each other deeply and are compatible in the most important ways. They share a common focus on emotional and spiritual growth, they both like healthy food and enjoy cooking together, they love each other's bodies, they communicate well with each other, they play and have fun together, and they even work together in a successful business.

Most times they are harmonious, but when they are stressed and overworked in their business they start to get on each other's nerves. Minor situations and stressors now become a problem — they bicker, blame each other for the smallest practical things, doubt the whole relationship and start to take distance from each other. After several years of being in this painful pattern, it has changed. First of all, they have finally been able to diagnose the problem accurately — they fight when they are stressed out.

Now, they are aware when the tension level builds, they take time away from each other, do what each of them needs to do to cool out and nourish themselves and come back together when they feel more in touch with themselves again. Also, both of them have been practicing the tension relieving exercise we present at the conclusion of the chapter.

When we're tense, we can make small triggers that ordinarily wouldn't bother us into a big problem. When life circumstances, for whatever reason, bring us tension, we can easily become irritable, moody, and easily provoked. Then the little things that bother us about the other person can seem insufferable. We begin to react to a behavior that we normally would simply ignore.

For example, six months of the year, often for three months at a time, we are on the road in Europe leading workshops. Sometimes, we don't have a long break between seminars and we have to travel long distances in our car. Both of us become tired, and we know that at the end of a day of driving we can be very testy and reactive. Since we know and can both feel that our nerves are frayed, we take time to be with ourselves. The next morning, everything seems different. Even if we reacted to each other in the evening about something, in the morning, it seems trivial.

Another time, we were in Japan and between workshops, went to visit an amusement park outside of Tokyo. Feeling courageous, we took a ride on a box that drops fifty meters and stops abruptly. Then we took some rides on a roller coaster. I (Krish) have motion sickness, and after those three rides my nervous system felt "shot." On the way back home, I could feel the tension in my body, and that night I picked a fight with Amana for absolutely no reason. It seemed real while I was in it but in the morning when I woke up, I could not believe that I had been disturbed. Amana was hurt and perplexed but when I finally explained to her that I was disturbed simply because I was overwhelmed by the experience at the amusement park, she was relieved. Now, we can use this experience as an example in our workshops for how couples can find something to fight about simply because they went to an amusement park. (By the way, I wouldn't recommend someone who suffers from motion sickness to get into a box that drops out of the sky.)

Finding Your Resources

Resources are anything that brings you back to yourself, which gives you more inner space — something that helps you to relax, to feel the joy of living, to feel a connection to existence and to take distance from what brings tension or disturbance inside. Most people are easily affected by many things in life that they cannot avoid — by setbacks, failure, rejection or even the anticipation of failure or rejection. You can also easily feel overwhelmed by life's daily stresses — the pressures of time, finances, deadlines and so on. And when you are impacted by these things, you may feel overwhelmed, self-critical, irritable or despairing. You lose touch with what makes life worth living. This is when you need to call on your resources.

It's a bit like learning to change channels. When your needle inches toward the red zone, your nervous system is activated and your psyche is overwhelmed. Your mind may be sending you all sorts of negative messages. When you start to soothe yourself, your nervous system starts to settle and a new reality sets in. The voices in your head change and the agitation inside is replaced by more peacefulness and stillness. A resource is not a one shot deal. It is something that you cultivate over time and then it bears fruit. For some, it can be moving the body in some way — a physical activity such as jogging, a sport, dance, yoga and so on. Or it can be some creative endeavor such as art, music or dance. You might connect deeply with yourself while spending time in nature. The vibration of a natural setting can soothe your nervous system and help you to come back home.

Sometimes, to develop a resource to the point that it begins to have significant effect in your life, you need to put some energy and commitment into it. For instance, a woman participant was sharing that she suffered from frequent crippling depression lasting for days at a time and sometimes could not even get herself out of bed. When we asked her what she did in her life that brought her joy and increased energy, she mentioned a long list — riding horses, practicing yoga, tai chi and meditation and dancing. We suggested that perhaps she might try becoming less diversified and focusing on just one of these.

A year later, we met her again and asked her how things were. She told us with much excitement that she had followed our suggestion and began taking tai chi lessons twice and later three times a week. Now she was even teaching tai chi in her town. When we asked her about her depression, she said that it was so improved that she had stopped taking anti-depressants, and when she did become depressed, she would recover quickly. What helped her, she said, was that the tai chi had become like a long lost friend to her and was there for her all the time — and especially when she needed a lift.

Another participant who also was depressive and even suicidal at times had taken up fitness training and long-distance running. She told us that this new hobby of hers saved her life. She trained regularly for runs and felt how much she enjoyed the aliveness in her body, eating in a healthy way, and feeling so proud of herself that she was able to confront her fears.

In our experience, one of the most important resources is finding healthy and life affirmative routines such as regular exercise, putting vitalizing and nourishing food into your body and finding time to relax and be alone. These kinds of routines have a number of positive affects on your life.

Most of us have a part inside which feels positive and inspired by life and by the search for truth, love, and contentment. We also have another side that feels overwhelmed, despairing and feels like giving up. We have an energy inside which pulls us toward truth, toward light and toward greater love – of ourselves, others and life in general. But we also have an opposite energy inside which pulls us down — toward depression, sabotage and self-destruction.

As you become more accustomed to living in a way that brings more light, you become more conditioned to live in the positive flow of life. Healthy routines nurture your positive side and gradually make your negative side less and less powerful. They build momentum and help to keep you on track because your being and body become accustomed to being nourished.

When you feel stressed or depressed, these routines help you to change channels and return your life to greater flow. They also help you to overcome self-destructive addictive behaviors because you replace negative habits with positive ones. Your body lets you know which it prefers. It's like you are giving your body a chance to return to its natural rhythm and wisdom.

It also helps to surround yourself with loving and supportive people. Very often in our work we point out to clients how important it is in their healing to separate from those people who bring up their shame and shock. Instead, we suggest they find people who help them to discover their essence, their gifts and their beauty. Sometimes this is difficult. For example, Andrea was living at home partly because it was more practical financially. But she was subjecting herself to the same negative and depressive energy from her mother, and the judgmental and often angry energy from her father that she had experienced all her childhood. Being in this energy field, she found herself often depressed and without energy. She felt that if she moved out not only would she face financial hardship but she would also betray her mother, who needed her for emotional support. We encouraged her to feel the price she was paying by living at home. Eventually it would occur to her that the price was greater that the guilt of leaving her mother, and the fear of learning to make it on her own.

We have both been developing our resources for many years, but above all our main resource is meditation — taking time to go inside and be present to whatever comes up. Meditation, in our experience, is the process of learning to become an observer to your life — your breath, body sensations, emotions, thoughts, disturbances, joy — witnessing whatever is happening in the moment. This quality develops over time.

At this point in our lives, meditation no longer means simply the act of sitting silently, although we also do this quite regularly. It means making the slight effort to watch all the time. Normally, without inner space, when disturbance, emotion, pain or fear arises, we move habitually, automatically and unconsciously into some kind of reaction. As meditation deepens, it becomes easier to return to watching the breath and the body and rather than react automatically. Then it becomes easier to discover what the natural response to any situation might be. This slowly lifts you out of the disturbance and out of the compulsive reactions and brings you back home.

Sex Flourishes When You Are Feeling Fulfilled In Your Life

One of the biggest causes of difficulties in your relationships and particularly in your sex lives comes not from interpersonal problems but from causes external to the relationship. For instance, when you feel unfulfilled and frustrated in your lives and in your creative expression, your sex life will suffer and you may even find yourself taking out your frustrations in sex. Not only is this an inappropriate place to act out your unhappiness and your anger, it only makes you feel worse. It is far better to recognize the root of the problem and take steps to heal it.

Your sexuality also suffers when you look to your partner or to sex as a way of relieving your anxiety and inner disturbance. Healthy sexuality is not meant to be a place for relieving your tension but a way to give (and receive) love. It is important to recognize when you are using sex for this purpose and find other ways to relieve your anxiety. In essence, sexuality is best served when it becomes a place you go to, not from deficiency, but from overflow, not from wanting to take but from wanting to give and to share.

An Exercise for Relieving Stress and Anxiety

1. Notice when you are getting disturbed, anxious or stressed. (You may notice that you are speeding up, becoming irritable, that you are talking rapidly etc.)

2. Take some time to feel the disturbance, tension and anxiety in the body. (Shallow breath, heart rate faster, tense muscles, acid stomach, sore back?)
3. Notice how the disturbance affects how you think. (Obsessive and reoccurring thoughts, focusing obsessively on details?)
4. Notice how you normally react (act out) from the disturbance. (Anger, blame, collapse, giving up, moving even faster?)
5. Now, take some time, if you can, to sit down, close our eyes and take five gentle deep breaths. Then, focus your attention as the breath becomes normal again, keeping your eyes closed. Ten minutes of this exercise can be enough to change your nervous system.
6. As you allow yourself to feel the tension, disturbance or anxiety, open your palms and give it up to existence. (And perhaps say to yourself, "Rather than fighting with this, I accept it and surrender it up to existence."

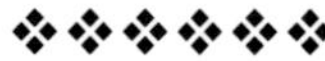

Chapter 12
"What Does It Mean to Communicate?" Learning How to Talk to Each Other

Recently, we were doing some work with a couple who were struggling in their relationship. They had been together for twelve years and had two children. It seemed that they fought about everything — about raising their children, about sex, about finances, and about where and when to go on vacations. The woman complained that her husband was too lenient and blamed him for their teenage daughter spending time with "the wrong crowd." She felt he was too aggressive in sex, did not share with her about their financial situation, and always wanted to vacation where he could play golf. He in turn complained that she did not really listen to her children, that she never initiated sex, that she was irresponsible with money and wanted to go to boring places on vacation.

Given that scenario, one would ask naturally wonder why they were still together. But strangely enough, they still loved each other and had much in common. The problem was that they could not communicate. They could not listen to each other. Whenever they tried to talk about things, they invariably would end up yelling at each other and one of them would either storm away or hang up the phone in frustration. But there is every possibility that these two can learn to talk and listen to each other. What was missing are some simple tools.

In our experience, the most helpful element for loving communication is a sincere desire to connect.

> *That means learning to listen to our beloved from the heart, becoming aware of and willing to feel our own fears and to expose ourselves without blame and wanting to be right.*

A while ago we were called in to arbitrate between two men friends who were having conflict. They worked together as therapists and one of them was renting space from the other who was running a small therapy center. As their grievances with each other came out, it became obvious to us that they both had valid reasons to be upset, hurt and angry with the other. However, one of them was unable to listen. Each time his friend tried to explain why he was hurt, he interrupted to defend himself and explain why he was right.

In the end, we gave up on trying to help them to resolve the conflict because there was not a mutual willingness to listen. The man who defended himself compulsively wasn't willing to own his side of the story and see that his friend also had justifiable reasons for being hurt. Without a shared intention to take each other in and listen, the conflict could not resolve.

Often, you may think that just because you are talking (or shouting) at each other, that you are communicating. It isn't true. To communicate, there has to be some part of you willing to listen. Most of us never learned to listen because we were not listened to as a child. I (Krish) know from my childhood, that I stopped sharing myself at an early age, although it wasn't until being in therapy much later that I recognized the reason. It didn't feel right to share because I was given advice and opinions instead of feeling listened to and taken in. I became allergic to advice and opinions (unless of course I asked for them) and still am. I wanted someone to listen, not try and fix me or direct me.

When I look back at my childhood environment, I can see that there were a lot of people talking but seldom communicating. In fact, there is a pattern in my family which I can still observe today of people thinking that they know what is best for someone else. When we grow up in an environment where people don't listen to each other, we never learn what it means to communicate.

What is communication, after all? It's two people exchanging information with each other. You have communicated when, afterwards, you know more about the other person — more about his or her feelings, thoughts, perspective and inner world. But communication becomes a challenge when it is with someone you are intimate with. It's hard to reach your partner when you are so emotional and fearful of not being heard or taken in that you can neither listen nor express yourself in a way that helps the other person to understand. You may have become so hurt and resentful, that you are not communicating, you are venting. Venting is usually attacking. Attacking generates counter attack and then instead of communication, you have war. But both may think you are communicating.

Over the years of being together, we've learned a few things about communicating — pretty important things. Here they are:

1. Emotions often don't express themselves in a way that helps the other person to hear us. They often wish to attack, blame or punish the other person and provoke defensiveness, hurt and resentment. Also, emotions don't listen well. They motivate you to defend and prove that you are right. It is seldom easy to communicate when we are emotionally involved with someone because emotions don't have ears. They only have mouths.

   In other words, when you are emotional, you can become obsessive about getting your point across and are much less interested in listening to the other person's point. When you are in an intimate relationship, you're going to be provoked over and over again. You want to be understood, respected, treated lovingly and sensitively, taken in, appreciated and loved unconditionally. You want to receive the kind of sex we long for. The list goes on and on. When you're emotional, you may be able to express yourself but that does not mean you are communicating. It is only once we have found some distance from the emotional storm that communication can happen.

> *In order to communicate, it helps to understand when we are taken over by our emotions and expressing or listening from that space. And it helps to understand the difference between when we are expressing ourselves like an emotional child and when we have some centeredness and composure.*

It is not that you are wrong or bad for venting, but it is important to understand that the emotional child in you does not communicate, she or he vents. *So, when you are emotional and disturbed, wait until you have cooled down and collected yourself before you attempt to communicate*

2. In an intimate relationship, you naturally project your unmet childhood needs on your partner and become upset when they are not met. However, your partner is not responsible to meet these needs. Until you become aware of your projections, you will contaminate your efforts to communicate in a mature way with childish expectations. *For intimacy to work, discover what and when you consciously or unconsciously project on your partner and own it back.*

   In an intimate relationship, you naturally project on your partner your sensitivities of being disrespected. When this sensitivity is triggered, you react automatically, habitually and unconsciously. *It greatly aids communication when you become aware of your sensitivities based on your childhood history of invasions.*

> *Often, when two people enter a love relationship — or any intimate relationship for that matter — they are not aware of how much they are going to get provoked, how easily and unconsciously they will project their needs on each other or be disrespectful of each other. That's why we strongly encourage people to become aware how their wounds may sabotage their love relationships. We know that inner work can*

sometimes feel tedious and without results. But hang in there! If you are sincerely committed to becoming more conscious human beings, there comes a time when your past no longer sabotages your efforts to create deep and sustained love in your life.

With these insights in mind, we would like to present some specific tools and guidelines for conscious communication.

a. *Are You Sharing to Communicate or to Vent?*
It may be healthy and important to vent your frustrations, hurts and anger. But don't mistake it for communication. Communication means having a mindset that you would like to give information about yourself but also receive information about the other person. It means that you not only would like to talk but also to listen, to set yourself aside and be open to feel and listen to your partner. If your intention is to try to convince your partner that you are right and they are wrong, this is not going to be communication. When you are emotional, it is natural to blame and try to make the other person feel wrong. But the chances are high that you will walk away feeling even more frustrated. When you are blaming, you are not being vulnerable and when your partner feels blamed, it also causes him or her to close.

b. *Are You Protected or Vulnerable?*

We ask this question because when you are aware of the difference between being vulnerable and being protected, you can understand the response and outcome you receive. Communication happens when you are vulnerable. Fighting and distance happens when you are protected. You usually receive the same kind of energy you are giving out. It is important to know what you are bringing to the table with the other person because this will determine the outcome. Protection has a certain feeling. It makes you tense, tight, held back or aggressive, guarded, suspicious, expecting and focused on the other person. Vulnerability feels differently. It feels more insecure, vulnerable and wanting to connect with the other person. Your attention is with yourself and with what you are feeling. It is not focused on getting something from or trying to change the other person.

When you feel hurt, the natural and customary reaction is to be in protection — to attack or to withdraw. But when you react in this way, you sabotage communication. Once you cool down a bit and allow yourself to feel and show the hurt to your partner, then communication can happen. The other person may not be ready to meet you with their vulnerability. You may need to wait. When both of you are not open to be vulnerable, it is a time to connect with the resources and wait for a time when a meeting is possible. If you are expecting that the other person is sensitive and open to you when you are ready, then you are still in protection — and you get protection back.

c. *Do You Have The Intention to Listen?*

Because most of us haven't been taught how to listen, it is not likely to come automatically. You need a specific conscious intention to listen. In order to listen, you have to make a conscious inner shift away from your emotions and neediness toward a space that is receptive and open. At the end of the chapter, we provide a simple exercise for conscious communication. (Again as we mentioned in an earlier chapter, we are indebted to the work of Harville Hendricks, mentioned in the references, from which we have loosely modeled this exercise.)

Listening takes practice. We recently tried this technique in a workshop with a couple who were having sexual problems. They were so emotional and hurt that when one spoke, the other continually interrupted, and as their sharing continued they both became increasingly heated and despairing. They both felt that they could never get their sexual needs met because the other person was not willing to change or even understand their feelings. They could recognize how emotional they were and how difficult it was to listen when the emotional barometer was rocketing to such high levels. It helped them to see that they were both reenacting old and painful patterns and to see that the roots of these patterns came from early life traumas.

It becomes easier to listen when you recognize how you're sabotaging your communication with your emotions and feel the panic behind your needs and fears. The next step, whenever possible, is to communicate the needs and fears from a place of vulnerability.

d. *What Are My Partner's Fears and Needs Right Now?*

In some ways, this point is included in all the three previous ones but it is so fundamental for communication that it deserves to be mentioned specifically. When we love someone, it doesn't mean that we have to attend to and satisfy the needs of the other person. But love does mean to open up to and feel his or her needs, fears and pain, to understand her or him more deeply and to take the other person into your heart.

Love presents us with an opportunity to transcend our narcissism, to get past our habitual focus on ourselves and learn to be present to another person.

This does not mean that you need to give up your own life, your own interests, or to rescue the other person from his or her fears. But it does mean that you are no longer thinking only in terms of yourself. Your thinking and your feeling includes your partner — how does he or she feel, what are his or her sensitivities, fears, longings, preferences, habits and idiosyncrasies. Your biggest challenge comes when you're triggered. That is when your love is tested because it is much easier to be loving when your buttons are not pushed. To keep your heart open even when you're afraid that your needs are not being met is a true test of love.

We have worked with Leo and Sylvia for several years. During this time, their relationship has been stormy. But partly what enabled them to stay together was that when they took time away from their fighting, they had great sex together. Energetically, they were well suited for each other. Both are passionate, intense, intelligent and good-hearted people. Both are quite successful in their respective careers and both have a deep willingness to grow and learn to love. Their sex life reflected this energetic compatibility. But when they spent other time together, boy, did they fight!

He felt invaded by her neediness and her demands that he listen to her and attend to her. She was physically abused by her father and, as a result, was hyperkinetic, hyper-talkative and extremely emotional. He was abused by an overprotective, domineering and possessive mother. When he felt overwhelmed by his wife, he would threaten to leave the relationship — and that only made her panic worse. But in spite of the high drama of their relating, they had a clear intention to treasure the love between them and learn to listen to each other.

We guided them in this simple technique of sharing and listening to each other's fears and hurts. His was being overwhelmed by her anxiety and not giving him the space to take distance from her when he needed to, which was quite similar to what he experienced as a child. Hers was the constant fear that he would find her too much and leave him just as had happened in her childhood. As they listened, they were both deeply touched by each other, and it opened them to feel the love that they felt for each other.

e. What Are My Fears and My Hurt?

The last question is in some ways the deepest and most significant. Whenever you are disturbed, whenever you are emotional, there is fear and hurt underneath. When your focus is not on discovering the fear and the hurt, on feeling it and on exposing it, your communication goes awry.

Unacknowledged, unfelt and unexposed hurt and fear is the saboteur of communication. When we react from hurt and fear, we make communication difficult because we are in a state of panic and from that space, push away the other person.

Your hurt is usually from either feeling misunderstood, deprived of love and attention, or feeling abandoned, unsafe or disrespected. If you examine this list, most likely you will find the source of your hurt and your fear. Hurt and fear cause you panic and when you are under the spell of panic, your main concern is not communication, it is creating safety for yourself or hurting the other person back. Once you become aware of this, even if you have reacted from panic, you can cool off and make a sincere effort to communicate.

Remember, the purpose of conscious communication is to deepen the love and the connection between you. It's not your nature to attack, punish, berate or prove to the other person that you are right. It's not in your nature to live in conflict or in resentment. But when you don't make a continual effort to stay connected and to communicate in a mature way, it is natural that hurt and distance grows. By following these simple steps, you're allowing the heart to take over again, the love to flow again and the relationship to keep deepening as it is meant to do. In short, communication happens when you have some distance from your fears and when you take in the feelings, fears and hurt of your partner.

A Simple Technique for Conscious Communication

Step 1. Become aware when you feel hurt, angry, and/or resentful or if your heart has closed to the other person. (If you are pulling away from the other person, don't let it pass, pretending that it doesn't matter because the distance will only get bigger. Make a decision to communicate.)

Step 2. If you feel hurt, angry or resentful, take some time to be with yourself. Time will often soften the charge. (Feel that your connection with this person is important for you. Go inside and feel if you have been invasive or disrespectful in some way. Take some time to feel your hurt and see if you can put this hurt into words.)

Step 3. Now, go to the other person and say that there is something important that you would like to express. Ask him or her if he or she has the space to listen. (If not, ask him or her to tell you when would be a good time because it is important. If there is no willingness to communicate at all, seek help from a professional or friend.)

Step 4. If there is a willingness to communicate, take ten minutes (precisely) to express yourself. You can begin by saying, "I felt hurt or upset when you…" (And be precise.) (Make an effort to talk about your feelings from your heart without blaming, attacking or analyzing the other person.) During those ten minutes, the other person simply listens. (At any time, if you as the listener feel like it is too much, you can say, "Wait, I just need some time to take this in.")

Step 5. Once you have expressed your hurt, the listener can say from their heart, "I hear you and I understand." (Listener — resist the temptation to defend yourself.)

Step 6. Now you, the listener, can take ten minutes to express yourself, following the same guidelines of the person who expressed himself or herself initially.

Step 7. You, the new listener, will respond by saying from your heart, "I hear you and I understand."

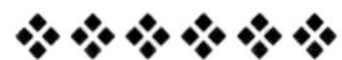

Chapter 13
"It's All About Connection." Living and Making Love in the "Love Current"

The experience of love is a world unto itself. It's as though love exists in a parallel world to the one that most of us are familiar with — the jungle world of competition, judgments, feeling inferior or superior, pressure, speed, power games and so on. This different world of love we call "the love current." It is heartfelt, gentle and flowing, it takes some inner work to find it and once you are in it, with yourself and/or with another person, it brings a deep sense of inner peace — as if something inside falls into place. This is your natural state of being, and finding it feels like coming home.

In the love current, shame and shock can arise, but you have the inner space to feel, accept and even love that part of you which holds these feelings. You also have more space to allow your intimate partner to be in shame or fear with compassion and without judgment. In this environment, these feelings and the sense of separation from yourself and from another pass more quickly. In the jungle world, shame, fear and shock can be devastating because you are already in a state of feeling separate and in judgment.

Finding Your Way Back to the Love Current

You leave the love current when your wounds are triggered and you react with blame, judgment, revenge, control, manipulation or isolation. In such moments, connecting with feeling and exposing your fear helps you to reenter or stay in the love current. When you leave the love current, it is extremely painful because you suddenly feel a separation and a disconnection from yourself and from your partner. Naturally you want to do everything possible to get back again. But your panic to return to the love current often makes it harder to find your way back. Sometimes there is nothing to do but wait and allow your heart and the love to come back. Most of the time, the love has not gone, it just feels gone because it is covered with hurt, fear and pain.

However, when you have made the commitment to nourish love and trust and to work through difficult times, it builds a foundation to be able to move more quickly out of the jungle and back to the love current. The effort you have put in to honor love pays off.

> *When we speak about love, we're not talking about an expansion of the heart that we may be able to feel in casual sexual connections. We're referring to the depth that develops only when we've nourished the flower of love in a long-term relationship that has gone through the trials of facing fear and shame and overcoming power games.*

Sex Can Test You to Stay in the Love Current

When you're in the love current, sex becomes truly "making love." Having sex while not being in the love current is just sex. When you're in the love current, there's a natural longing to come closer to the one you love, to feel and deepen the connection. And when you're in the love current, you can bring the bodies together to make love even when one or both of you are not "turned on." You simply want to be together.

However, sometimes sex presents you with some challenges to remain in the love current with your partner. If nothing has disturbed the love current, when you're making love, the sexual energy can flow easily and spontaneously. You may feel deeply fulfilled and nourished. But sometimes the situation is not so free of complications. One of you can be touching your shame and your shock and not be able to open or to communicate freely or spontaneously. Or you may feel inhibited or insecure or resentful with your partner. Or you may discover that there is a disharmony in the way each of you would like to make love. Or you may simply need new tools for making love in a way that suits both of you.

When two people encounter disharmony in the way that they want to make love, the love is tested. When one person starts to encounter unexplainable reactions in the body and finds it hard to explain them to him or herself and even harder to explain them to his or her partner, the love is tested. When one person feels that he or she would like to move out of conventional loving making toward more meditative sexuality while the other person wants passion and excitement, the love is tested. When one person is rejecting lovemaking but doesn't know why, the love is tested. When the love is deep and the longing to be in the love current is strong, there is a possibility that you can pass through these tests and even grow through them.

We have known Stan and Elizabeth for a long time. They were having tremendous difficulties in their sex life because they wanted to make love in different ways. Stan wanted hotter and more passionate sex with a lot of activity, while Elizabeth wanted it to be slow and more passive. They were at the point of breaking up because they were fighting about this issue continually — even though they still loved each other and had two young children.

To stay together, they were willing to do whatever they could and were open to learning what could help them. We had worked earlier with their emotional issues but the problem was not that. Their problem was simply that they needed to find a new way of making love. We referred them to a couple who are acquaintances of ours, who teach a lovemaking technique that we will describe shortly. It helped them to learn to be sensitive to each other, to allow them both to feel safe, and to enable the love current to take over.

In the Love Current, It's All About Connection

Sexual intimacy basically means that while making love, each person becomes equally sensitive and attuned to both him or herself and to the other person. When you are in the love current, there is no longer an agenda or an idea that sex has to be a certain way to be "good." With this kind of sensitivity, it becomes safer to feel your vulnerability and even your trauma if it arises. The space between you opens to embrace the fears and insecurities. Sex at this level is no longer a taking or using the other to reach orgasm. It is a giving for both people. Paradoxically, with this kind of sensitivity, there is also space for a different kind of passion and intensity to arise. This is what we call "level three sex."

In "level three sex," the love that has built up between you embraces whatever comes up when you make love. There develops a willingness, even if it is hard, to be with to feel and to share whatever is arising. As soon as disharmony arises, you make an effort to communicate without blame. And you make that effort because your highest priority is to find a way to return to the love current. The paradox is, and we've experienced this time and again, when the love embraces shame, shock, dysfunction and fear, very often even these feelings diminish and sometimes disappear altogether.

Finding New Ways of Making Love

In "level three sex," there is no "right" way to make love, but you may discover that something does change in your lovemaking. As love deepens, you also want more depth while making love — more connection. You may also experience that you have a longing for more silence and less doing. When you are in the love current, it is immensely nourishing just to feel the energy of love that is flowing between you and surrounding you. It is easier to feel this when you become more silent and less active – feeling the breath coming and going within each of you, feeling the subtle contact of the two bodies being together and the sensitivity that arises in the genitals when you are being more passive.

As we mentioned earlier, when we began our relationship, we learned a way of making love that was radically different from what we had known before. We took a course that taught the lovemaking principles of sexuality teacher Barry Long. His teachings are quite radical and beautiful. He claims that lovemaking has been contaminated with doing and addiction to excitement. In his view, the way in which most people have been conditioned to make love — with in and out movement, orgasm and driven by excitement — the vagina has become infected with male aggression and violence.

In this way, it has learned lovemaking that is foreign to its nature. According to Barry, its nature is to open and receive a penis that is not aggressive and goal-oriented, but sensitive, loving and present. In his view, when we make love in a way which is more still and focused on connection rather than excitement and orgasm, we naturally become acutely present to ourselves and to the other and stay connected through eye contact, body awareness and presence to the moment.

In the course, we learned a very specific method for making love that followed this teacher's principles. The approach is described in more detail and with much greater competence in the references we provide (Barry Long, *Making Love*, and Diana Richardson, *The Heart of Tantric Sex*). But we would like to mention a bit about it, particularly how we have adopted it. In this method, anything that stimulates excitement is discouraged. Instead, a couple brings the bodies together and finding a comfortable position for each person, the man, in a relaxed way, comes inside the woman and simply rests. The emphasis is to avoid repetitive movement, maintain eye contact, and relax with the breathing, making a commitment to stay present and occasionally sharing what each one is experiencing in the body.

After a time, it is okay to include some gentle side-to-side movement (rather than in and out movement) just to keep up a slight amount of sexual stimulation. Slight sexual stimulation is used simply to help maintain an erection but it is not so important if the penis is totally hard. In fact, when it is slightly soft, it can become more sensitive. Also, orgasm is discouraged. If it happens, it is not a problem, but since the teaching is to learn to move away from the addiction to excitement, orgasm is basically not part of the practice.

We no longer practice the technique as it was originally described to us because we shy away from any technique or method and prefer to flow with however we feel in the moment. Yet this approach has become the basis of how we make love. While it is not our intention (nor even our expertise) in this book to teach this particular method — or any lovemaking method for that matter — we have found that learning an alternative way of making love which focuses on connection without moving automatically into excitement can be extremely helpful for many reasons.

- It deepens lovemaking and connection. Excitement can often be a way of running away from depth of intimacy. When you take time to connect, you begin to touch each other in your deepest core.
- It also is a way for couples to make love when there is fear or insecurity because it slowly enables the fear to subside as the trust and sensitivity grows. Taking time to relax and allowing and accepting for fears and insecurity or whatever else surfaces in the lovemaking creates trust.
- It also reminds you to stay in touch with your own and your partner's body and needs.
- Finally, it helps men from losing too much energy through orgasm (which is really great for me (Krish) since it leaves me more energy for playing tennis which is my greatest passion in the world - second only to making love with Amana but a very close second).

Also, in the course of learning to make love in this non-active way, I (Krish) discovered something profound for myself. Feeling the love current while we are making love has replaced the need for me to have the sometimes compulsive and habitualized orgasm. I noticed that previously I was somewhat addicted to orgasm and even made love with a subtle anticipation of coming. I still enjoy passion — Amana's and mine — but it isn't a compulsion anymore.

There is also something else to mention that we have experienced. When you move toward non-active sex, it involves a period of adjustment. You may find the lovemaking "boring" initially because you are used to excitement. But when you feel the love current, it fills the space of boredom. In fact, often non-activity gives greater space to feel the love current and the connection between you. It is as though you are opening to a different kind of nourishment than you are used to from the high intensity of excitement. But it is a kind of nourishment that in many ways feels deeper and more satisfying.

A couple we have worked with were attempting to make love in a more non-active way but were encountering difficulties. He would start out by going through his usual maneuvers of turning her on, but when he entered her with the intention of slowing down and relaxing together, he would come. Then he felt so much shame that he went into his cave and could not communicate.

She said, "I feel that I am getting mixed messages. I am not sure if he wants to have hot sex or to make love in this new way. Once we both get turned on, it is natural that we move into the old way. Also, when he comes so fast, I feel a bit betrayed."

We asked him, "How is it for you to make love without getting all turned on?"

"I don't really feel like a man then," he answered.

"How about cooling yourself down before you go inside her?" we suggested. "It's not so easy to hold back from coming when both of you are hot."

"I never thought about that."

"Making love without the customary excitement can bring up your shame and insecurities of not being 'man enough,' but that is part of the experience," we said. "Do you feel that this might be worthwhile for you?"

He hesitated.

She said to us, "I have really longed for him to share these parts of himself. I think that it would bring us much closer together."

"And anyway," she said to him, "you don't have to prove yourself as a man to me. I like it much better when we just connect with each other. Then I can feel our connection and that is more than enough for me because I love you."

Conventional Hot Sex Can Be Re-traumatizing

Moving away from excitement can create a greater amount of safety. With hot sex, it's easier to feel traumatized, particularly if you have a history of sexual trauma. Not only can it cause people to have painful flashbacks but you can also become re-traumatized with the speed and intensity of hot sex. Then your body becomes constricted and you may become afraid of making love altogether. The people we have worked with who have entered into the vulnerability/trauma layer in sex have all said the same thing. If their partner slows down and becomes deeply sensitive and respectful of their fears, they can slowly — very slowly — feel safe enough to open again. And, surprisingly, they can even return to hot sex with more enjoyment and deeper, more nourishing orgasms than they ever had before.

Andrew and Manuela, a couple we worked with recently, were faced with precisely this situation. She started by saying, "I am feeling intense fear coming up whenever we make love or even anticipate making love."

He said, "If I am honest, I am feeling impatient that she is so afraid. I feel that it is a power trip on her part, that she is just pushing away my 'maleness' because she doesn't want me to 'be in my power' and she doesn't want to lose control. Furthermore, to make love in a way which was slower and in which I can't move as I want to feels emasculating to me and I feel controlled by her fears."

As the session progressed, she told us that she was uncovering a sexual-abuse story that she did not know about previously.

"Yes," he said, "but I can't understand how something that happened so long ago could affect you today. And why now? How come you have so much fear all of a sudden? You used to be so wild and uninhibited."

We explained, "What you are both experiencing is really common. Often, the body and actual visual memories of trauma come up after we have gone deeper into intimacy with someone. Now, Manuela is connecting with her sexual trauma because your relationship is deepening and that is affecting how she can make love. Prior to that, she had been overriding herself and her body sexually which is often the case when we have been abused. But as she becomes more sensitive and uncovers deeper layers in therapy, her vulnerability and fears are surfacing."

As he listened, he softened visibly and finally said, "It's good for me to hear this explanation. And I can see that she needs a different approach to lovemaking now."

We added, "It might help if you imagine that your penis is becoming an instrument of love, one that is even healing her and her vagina with its sensitivity, presence and love — your 'mission possible,' if you choose to accept it. And take it as a deep learning and growing for you."

"It's a big leap for me but I will try. I love Manuela. Right now I don't know if I can tolerate not being able to make love the way I want to and not being able to be in my sexual energy."

Manuela also had her challenge, which was to continue healing her trauma in her therapy and workshops, and communicate her process with him. We ended with both of them feeling relieved that at least they knew what they were facing.

When we describe this approach in our work, we focus not so much on the specifics of the technique but on slowing down, focusing on connection, bringing more sensitivity to the lovemaking and on getting away from the stress of performance and goal orientation. When we talk about it, the women almost universally find themselves very attracted. Most say that this is what they have always wanted, that this slowing down, being more in tune with each other and focusing on connecting rather than coming is really what they want. Some men also found it a relief. But as a rule, the men have more difficulty adjusting to sex without the heat, excitement, intensity and passion and orgasm as an end result. There isn't a right way or a wrong way. The softer way is not better than the hot way. It is just different.

> *But when we move into hot, excited sex without first connecting deeply with our partner and feeling the energies melt together, then it is very easy to drift away and not be present in the body. If we take the time to first connect, then it might happen that hot passionate sex arises. And when it arises on it's own rather than programmed, it has a totally different feeling to it.*

Honoring the Needs of Togetherness

Love constantly causes you to face new challenges, new hurdles, and new tests. One of those hurdles is that your sexuality most often will have to adjust to the needs of the togetherness. If you put your needs before the love, you will have trouble facing these obstacles.

In love, the highest goal is not your individual needs but the needs of the togetherness. That does not mean that you have to deny your needs. But when they conflict with what is necessary to keep the love flowing, then you have to ask yourself which is more important to you. It becomes a choice — the choice between going with the love and going with yourself.

We cannot say what is right for someone when faced with this challenge. There is usually a deeper learning for everyone involved if you go for love, but you have to feel that this is what you want and that it was right for you. You have to feel deeply inside that it is your choice and your learning, not that you are doing it for your partner.

In every relationship, it takes intention to stay in the love current. Not every relationship is meant to last the long haul, that's for sure. But none will survive the tests without a clear understanding from both sides that love takes work. When you choose the love option, love will guide you. It has a mystery of its own which has its own momentum and ultimately helps us to come home.

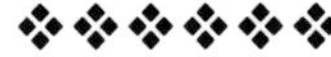

Conclusion

From Sex to Love
Embracing, Enjoying and Transcending Passion

When you approach intimacy and sexuality as a spiritual path, it begins with embracing your passion and ends with transcending passion. Sexual passion is life energy, and if you repress it, it isn't going to move into higher spiritual states. Repression leads to fantasies about sex, sexual games or perversions, and obsession with pornography. Or the sexual energy gets diverted towards something else like food, drugs, work, power or money.

Our spiritual master once mentioned that the essence of sexual desire and passion is a longing to attain something through the body which the body and sex cannot give us. The longing itself is beautiful, but the most that sexual desire and passion can lead to is a short glimpse of what we are seeking. Eventually, you may want more than that — a more sustaining experience of a higher state of consciousness. Sex can give you that when you begin to transform it into a deeply loving meditative experience.

Lovemaking that focuses on connection rather than performance or orgasm is the flowering of love.

A friend of ours told us recently that when he makes love with his girlfriend, he hardly ever comes anymore, yet he feels differently the whole day. He feels connected to her and to himself and he feels as though his body is humming inside. We both thought that this was a beautiful way of describing how sex can nourish us, and this is also our experience. Each intimate meeting deepens and strengthens the love current and the connection.

In these pages, we have been exploring what we have found helps a couple to keep their sexuality vibrant and nourishing. The single most important ingredient for sex to keep working between two people is to keep the love alive. When love is there, our sexual differences, vulnerabilities, insecurities and fears can be resolved. Our first responsibility, then, is to be vigilant in resolving conflicts that arise and making every effort to understand and be sensitive to each other.

Hopefully some of the keys we have provided for nourishing the flower of love can help in this respect. It also helps to be aware that sex is an area where your vulnerability — your fears and shame — will arise more readily than any other area in life. But when love guides the way, lovers can be aware when this happens and can be loving toward themselves and their partner when it does.

When love is the priority, then rules, ideals and standards don't work. Love always goes with the flow. If it's hot, great! Connect in passion. If it's not, great! Connect in greater stillness. But stay connected. It's all too easy, when stress, resentment and unresolved conflicts build, to escape into regarding your love partner, even your intimate partner, as a sexual object. You can get turned on and have orgasm without dealing with any underlying issues. But when you truly love, you also feel the pain of taking this route. And the pain guides you back home, back toward repairing the connection and getting back to the love current.

When you stay connected in love and make this the gold standard for your sexuality, your lovemaking brings the nectar of the gods. It is nourishing beyond comparison. It is easily one of the greatest gifts that life can offer and that is our passion and motivation for sharing what we have shared in this book. We also know, from our experience, that it takes commitment, perseverance and a constant willingness to "keep the house clean" — in other words, to clear up anything which disturbs the love current.

Sometimes it is not so easy to know what disturbs the love flow or how to deal with it effectively, but if there is love, there is a way.

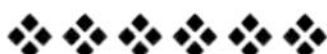

Selected References

Anderson, Susan The Journey from Abandonment to Healing — Surviving Through and Recovering From, the Five Stages that Accompany the Loss of Love Berkeley Books, 2000

Carlton, Randolph S. (Editor) Treating Sexual Disorders, Jossey-Bass 1996

Carnes, Patrick Don't Call It Love — Recovery from Sexual Addiction, A Bantam Book 1992

Carnes, Patrick Out of the Shadows — Understanding Sexual Addiction, Hazeldon 2001

Deida, David It's A Guy's Thing Health Communications, Inc 1997

Henderson, Julie The Lover Within — Opening to Energy in Sexual Practice Station Hill Press 1987

Hendrix, Harville, Ph.D. Keeping the Love You Find — A Personal Guide Pocket Books1992

Kingma, Daphne Rose Coming Apart — Why Relationships End and How to Live Through the Ending of Yours Fawcett Crest 1987

Lerner, Rokelle Living in the Comfort Zone — The Gift of Boundaries in Relationships Health Communications, Inc 1995

Levine, Stephen and Ondrea Embracing the Beloved — Relationship as a Path of Awakening Anchor Books 1995

Mellody, Pia Facing Love Addiction — Giving Yourself the Power to Change the Way You Love Health Communications, Inc 1992

Osho, Intimacy — Trusting Oneself and the Other St. Martin's Griffin 2001

Osho, Sex Matters — From Sex to Super Consciousness St. Martin's Griffin 2002

Long, Barry Making Love — Sexual Love The Divine Way Barry Long Books 1984

Morin, Jack, Ph. D. The Erotic Mind – Unlocking the Inner Sources of Sexual Passion and Fulfillment Harper Perennial 1995

Peabody, Susan Addiction to Love — Overcoming Obsession and Dependency in Relationships Celestial Arts 1994

Plaut, S. Michael, Graziottin, Alessandra, and Heaton, Jeremy PW Sexual Dysfunction

Health Press, Oxford 2004

Richardson, Diana The Heart of Tantric Sex, A Unique Guide to Love and Sexual Fulfillment, O Books Alresford, Hants UK 2003

Robinson, Marnia Peace Between the Sheets — Healing with Sexual Relationships Frog Ltd. 2002

Stone, Hal Ph. D. and Sidra Ph. D. Partnering — A New Kind of Relationship New World Library 2000

Wincze, John P. and Carey, Michael P. Sexual Dysfunction — A Guide For Assessment and Treatment The Guilford Press 2001

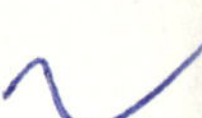

CPSIA information can be obtained at www.ICGtesting.com
Printed in the USA
BVOW07s1644010813

327443BV00003B/519/P